AMPLITUDE/PHASE PATTERNS IN DYNAMIC SCINTIGRAPHIC
IMAGING

DEVELOPMENTS IN NUCLEAR MEDICINE
Series editor Peter H. Cox

*Other titles in this series*

Cox, P.H. (ed.): Cholescintigraphy. 1981. ISBN 90-247-2524-0
Cox, P.H. (ed.): Progress in radiopharmacology 3. Selected Topics. 1982.
  ISBN 90-247-2768-5
Jonckheer, M.H. and Deconinck, F. (eds.): X-ray fluorescent scanning of the
  thyroid. 1983. ISBN 0-89838-561-X
Kristensen, K. and Nørbygaard, E. (eds.): Safety and efficacy of radiopharma-
  ceuticals. 1984. ISBN 0-89838-609-8

# Amplitude/phase patterns in dynamic scintigraphic imaging

**AXEL BOSSUYT**
**FRANK DECONINCK**

*Department of Nuclear Medicine*
*Vrije Universiteit Brussel*
*Brussels*
*Belgium*

1984 **MARTINUS NIJHOFF PUBLISHERS**
a member of the KLUWER ACADEMIC PUBLISHERS GROUP
BOSTON / THE HAGUE / DORDRECHT / LANCASTER
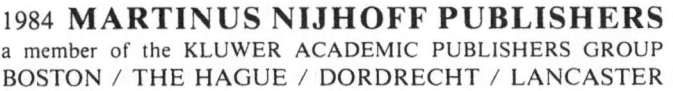

**Distributors**

*for the United States and Canada*: Kluwer Boston, Inc., 190 Old Derby Street, Hingham, MA 02043, USA
*for all other countries*: Kluwer Academic Publishers Group, Distribution Center, P.O.Box 322, 3300 AH Dordrecht, The Netherlands

**Library of Congress Cataloging in Publication Data**

Bossuyt, Axel.
   Amplitude/phase patterns in dynamic scintigraphic
imaging.

   (Developments in nuclear medicine)
   Includes index.
   1. Radioisotope scanning--Mathematics.  2. Image
processing--Digital techniques.  3. Inaging systems
in medicine.  4. Fourier transformations.  I. Deconinck, F.
II. Title.  III. Series.
RC78.7.R4B67 1984     616.07'575     84-4212
ISBN-13: 978-94-009-6011-4                 e-ISBN-13: 978-94-009-6009-1
DOI: 10.1007/978-94-009-6009-1

**Copyright**

Foreword by A. Bertrand Brill, MD, PhD                                VII

Introduction                                                             1

1.  The  temporal Fourier transform as a general approach to
    functional isotopic imaging.                                         9

2.  Amplitude/phase imaging of transient phenomena: superior
    cavography.                                                         20

3.  Regional breathing patterns studied by dynamic transmis-
    sion scintigraphy and the temporal Fourier transform.              29

4.  Amplitude/phase  images as a temporal condensate of  the
    averaged cardiac cycle.                                            43

5.  Clinical evaluation of amplitude/phase analysis for  the
    assessment of regional wall motion disturbances.                   56

6.  Non-invasive  assessment of the proximal stenoses of the
    main coronary arteries by means of exercise radionuclide
    ventriculography.                                                  70

7.  Functional dissimilarity between anterior and posterior
    ventricular walls during acute myocardial infarction.             86

8.  Scintigraphic visualisation of the effect of conduction
    disturbances  on  the mechanical events of  the  cardiac
    cycle.                                                            101

9.  Parametric imaging and temporal contrast enhancement for
    the visualisation of time patterns.                               110

10. Radionuclide  indices  of cardiac function  related  to
    structural ventricular disorders.                                 121

Conclusions                                                           138

Color plates                                                          145

Index of Subjects                                                     157

FOREWORD

By A. Bertrand Brill, MD, PhD.


The value of nuclear medicine imaging procedures, de-
rives from the physiological and biochemical functional
information they provide non destructively on living systems. The development of improved instrumentation capable of
imaging the body in three spatial dimensions (tomography),
and a fourth temporal dimension has been facilitated by the
rapid development in computing technologies. These in turn
have made it feasible to develop and use new short-lived
tracers for the study of processes with fast time constants.
Together, these innovation now make it possible to analyze
biological kinetics in vivo. The ability to view those
images and to assimilate these data in a meaningful way
poses many challenges. Key to the analysis of such data is
the development and use of appropriate mathematical models
to reveal essential features of the biological system, its
alteration in disease, or its response to interventions of
various kinds (exercise, drugs, etc...), for each individual
subject studies.

Modeling of vascular transients is simplified by the
possibility of measuring at multiple sites along perfused
channels, and well established methods exist for such analyses. Organ kinetics, using models of processes that inter-
vene between the inflow and outflow, are also used in diagnostic and metabolic research. The task of modeling and
analyzing projections of organs and interpreting function in
sub elements of complex structures with multiple overlapping

cross connections is extremely complex, and has yet to be solved.

This book presents an approach which utilizes a simple model in which each local picture element (pixel) or volume element (voxel) is fit along the time line by a smoothed curve. The curve is fit by sums of sine and cosine terms using a Fourier transform, and the phase and amplitude of the first harmonic are displayed. The utility of this approach has been well accepted in the area to which it has been applied most widely - i.e. nuclear cardiology and analysis programs to produce such results are now available on most nuclear medicine computer systems. The authors pioneered in the development of these systems and have done an admirable job in describing the method and illustrating a number of different potentially important applications.

The first chapter provides an explicit, and yet intuitively clear description of the essential features of the method. The second chapter describes the use of the technique in analysis of a transient phenomenon - superior vena cavography - based upon first-pass tracer kinetics. Despite the fact that the data are noisy and only poorly fit by a sinusoid curve, the phase and amplitude images reveal flow pattern abnormalities in patients with thyroid enlargement and SVC obstruction brought out by neck flexion which are not as obvious in traditional $t_{max}$, and transit time images. The third chapter illustrates the use of the method in analysis of pulmonary transients, where respiratory-gated transmission patterns are shown to provide clear evidence of regional variations (phase and amplitude changes) which correlate with normal physiology and provide evidence of localized changes in patients with COPD. The role of different breathing and therapeutic maneuvres is illustrated and provides physiological confirmation of interest to pulmonary medicine. Whether these simple transmission-gated pulmonary studies provide similar patterns as revealed by the more complex radioactive gas ventilation studies, or radio-aerosol distributions remains to be determined.

As a prelude to the remaining chapters in the book which deal with nuclear cardiology applications, the authors compare the signal and noise content of phase/amplitude imaging with conventional functional images (stroke volume, ejection fraction) and show the improvement obtained by use of the temporal Fourier transform method. The small contribution of higher harmonics is shown to be negligible in terms of global power density criteria. Whether local information of importance can be extracted from the higher order shape analyses remains to be established. In any case, other means of attacking that problem in physiologic terms are worthy of continued attention.

The remaining chapters focus on the clinical testing of the phase and amplitude images and parameters in nuclear cardiology. A comparison of wall motion (WM) abnormalities is presented using contrast angiography as the gold standard. When only the diagnosis of normal vs abnormal wall motion is analyzed, the sensitivity and specificity of the radionuclide WM images is enhanced impressively.

Results in patients found to have coronary artery le-sions by X-ray coronary angiograms are presented which show an impressive score for their methodology - i.e. complete agreement on specificity and high sensitivity for the diag-nosis based on a abnormal rest or exercise study.

Studies in a large number of patients admitted to their coronary care unit with transmural myocardial infarction were conducted within 72 hours of admission and 8-12 days thereafter. Correlations of the lesion locations and the findings with the radionuclide studies are presented which have relevance to the efficacy of different means of acquiring the data (different views for different lesion locations). Like other investigators, they find that ejection fraction alone is not an adequate descriptor of infarction, and that quantitative analysis of asynchrony in wall motion is also needed. The next chapter follows logically in that conduction disturbances per se involving left and right bundle branch blocks are clearly distinguished on the basis of phase shifts.

The concluding chapters deal with the methodology and variations that may increase its range of application and enhance its utility. Given that higher order harmonics are not needed for preservation of the information in phase and amplitude images, they show that four images through a repetitive cycle are an adequate representation of the temporal variation observed in the nuclear cardiography studies. Thus, it becomes possible to gate in core, high resolution (128 x 128) images of dynamic processes in real time. This has real attraction for the routine application of these methods in busy clinics. Further, they show that it is possible to achieve temporal contrast enhancement by the use of background substraction techniques using the minimum value in each pixel as its individual baseline.

The last chapter in the book illustrates a variety of indices that can be derived from the gated nuclear cardiology studies. These parameters were classified using principle component analysis methods along with classical measures, such as blood pressure and heart rate data. A distinct separation between patients with triple vessel disease and anterior wall motion abnormalities was achieved from patients with posterior wall motion abnormalities. The different parameters that can be extracted from these images provide an interesting data set to test the utility of classification techniques for use in differentiating patients with different underlying abnormalities.

This remarkable book presents a comprehensive description of a method and a broad test of its applicability. It is the result of the collaborative efforts of a physician - Dr A. Bossuyt - and a physicist - Dr F. Deconinck - who together have significantly advanced a method and tested it in a rich set of applications. The book provides an example and a challenge to future workers in the field and deserves careful reading by scientists and physicians alike. The role of the method extends beyond nuclear medicine and deserves attention in the various digital imaging and tomography analysis procedures where large amounts of data are obtained and efficient methods are needed for their analysis and display.

A. Bertrand Brill, M.D., Ph.D.
Director, Medical Department
Brookhaven National Laboratory
Upton, Long Island,
New York 11973
U.S.A.

# INTRODUCTION

Conventional nuclear medicine procedures study the distribution of radiolabelled compounds (radiopharmaceuticals) in the body under physiological as well as under pathological conditions. Because of their ability to visualise and to quantify the distribution of radiopharmaceuticals within the body by means of external detectors, nuclear medicine techniques are basically non invasive and function oriented. The spatial variation of the tracer distribution in the field of view, or the change in distribution during a time interval are interpreted as representing specific physiologic or pathophysiologic processes. As compared to other diagnostic imaging techniques, the spatial resolution of scintigraphic images is rather poor, their temporal resolution is good.

Factors that will therefore determine the ultimate diagnostic value of a scintigraphic study include :
1. The specificity of the labelled compounds for the process under study,
2. The  resolution in time and space of the instrumentation, and its ability  of measuring quantitatively tissue activity concentrations,
3. The formulation  of  physiological or pathophysiological models from which the distribution of the tracer can be predicted.

While interpreting nuclear medicine data, the interrelations between these factors should permanently remain under consideration.

The generalised use of minicomputers has resulted in major advances in information processing in nuclear medicine imaging procedures. Central to this is image digitisation. The digitised image is stored and handled as a matrix, the size of which is usually limited to 64 x 64 (up to 256 x 256) picture elements (= pixels). Information processing in nuclear imaging can cover two fields. In the first place, image enhancement and image restoration techniques are used to improve the localisation in time and space of the detected signals e.g. the visual appearance of an image may be improved by the use of filtering techniques or tomographic reconstruction techniques may be applied to convert the original data to images better suited for visual analysis. On the other hand, digital image analysis is concerned with the extraction of quantitative information or with the extraction of more relevant functional parameters from the original images.

The visualisation of organ function using functional images in which the value of each picture element represents a measure for the functional integrity of that anatomical structure is essential to the development of nuclear medicine procedures. Examples of the display of organ function in the form of a visual image are as old as imaging in nuclear medicine. Functional mapping of organ systems may be achieved either by the development of more specific radiopharmaceuticals, or by computing more complex parameters using a functional model of the organ. Therefore 2 types of functional images are currently distinguished from each other (1).

1. Direct functional images in which some particular property of an intrinsic metabolite or radiopharmaceutical
   is used to image directly a metabolic pathway or the
   physiology of an organ.
2. Indirect or parametric images which involve the mathematical manipulation of a set of images in order to compute
   and display some more complex aspect related to the
   physiology of an organ.

Examples of direct functional images would be the use of
$^{131}$I to visualise the areas in the thyroid of greater or
lesser function, the use of ($^{18}$F)-2-fluoro-2-deoxyglucose to
study the metabolic state of brain or myocardium, the
visualisation of regional perfusion after injection of
labeled microspheres. Examples of parametric images may be
the ventilation/perfusion ratio images of the lungs, or the
regional ejection fraction images of the left ventricle.

Parametric functional images were originally introduced
in nuclear medicine as a method for effectively dealing with
the vast amount of data in a dynamic image series (2,3,4).
As such they represent a form of data compression,
representing in a single image the characteristics of the
temporal variations of activity in all the pixels of the
field of view. The detection of regions of a scene which can
be seen to change from frame to frame in a time series of
images has also been a subject of investigation in other
fields, not related to biomedical applications of image
processing. For instance in the field of remote sensing,
where correlation methods are used for the study of cloud
motion in weather satellite pictures (5) and for the
detection of regions of seasonal change in pictures returned
by various Mars missions. However, most image processing
techniques deal almost exclusively with spatial information
and not with the time information present in a dynamic

series of images. In biomedical imaging, as most
physiological events are the result of combinations of
spatial and temporal interactions, the time information is
of particular importance. Time information is available
among others in radioscopic, angiographic and echographic
procedures. In nuclear medicine the measurement of the time
sequence of the event as a parameter reflecting a
physiological process, is inherent to the tracer
methodology.

Different approaches can be used for the calculation of
the parameters to be represented in a functional image.
Pattern recognition methods such as factor analysis (6) or
principle component analysis calculate the parameters which
allow the best classification of images between a number of
categories. No a priori knowledge of a physiological model
for the function under study is therefore required.
Different renal and cardiac functional imaging procedures
have been proposed using this approach (7,8). The method
does not determine true physiological factors related to the
existence of an underlying physiological model. This limits
the interpretability of such procedures. However, because
factor analysis enables the gamma-camera measurements to be
described in relation to the unknown model and because it
furnishes a lower limit to the number of elementary
structures of the model, it can be applied with success as a
first approach to the analysis of the underlying
physiological model in different routine dynamic
scintigraphic studies (9,10).

An alternative approach relies upon some a priori
physiological model of the scintigraphic study to describe
the response function to the tracer administration (the
input).

Mathematically, 2 general techniques may be used for the description of the response to input function : Fourier analysis and the Green function method. The Green function method describes the input as an infinite series of successive impulses of varying amplitude and calculates the impulse response. This principle was successfully applied in nuclear medicine for the calculation of transit times in renograms and in cerebral blood flow studies (11,12). These applications were limited to the analysis of curves and provide only globalised information on regions of interest in the image series (e.g. hemispheres, kidneys). Fourier analysis considers the input function as the sum of an infinite number of harmonic functions of varying frequency, amplitude and phase and calculates the response function to a sinusoidal input.

The work presented here involves the application of a temporal Fourier transform (TFT) as a functional imaging procedure. The variations in count rate occuring during a given time interval in a dynamic series of scintigraphic images are analysed in order to visualise regional time patterns in terms of magnitude and timing of the count rate changes. Amplitude and phase of the fundamental frequency (1st harmonic) are computed and displayed on a pixel per pixel basis in appropriate color codes.

The application to scintigraphic image processing of a Fourier transform in the time domain originates from the demands for data processing of radionuclide ventriculography (13). The principle may well, however, be applied to other scintigraphic procedures. Radionuclide ventriculography involves the evaluation of ventricular performance by means of radioactive tracers that remain within the intravascular space during the period of study. Due to this lack of specificity of the tracer, quantification of hemodynamic parameters is almost exclusively determined by the possibilities of data processing. The approximation of the changes in ventricular count rate by a sinusoidal function was introduced by Schelbert (14) for the calculation of left ventricular ejection fraction from first pass angiocardiographic studies. The use of first harmonic amplitude and phase functional images to visualise which parts of an image showed periodic changes in activity synchronously with the heart frequency was first described at Ulm (15,16). At present due to its predominant role in parametric heart imaging, amplitude/phase analysis is considered as an essential requirement of software packages for nuclear cardiology (17). To major facts have contributed to this:

1. In terms of amplitude and phase, 2 main diagnostic problems, "extent of regional contraction" and "coordination of motion", can be solved by only one algorithm.
2. The introduction of temporal criteria such as phase shifts provides a computationally inexpensive tool for the quantitation of ventricular synchronism by means of phase distribution functions.

The guide-line in this monography is the chronological evolution of our insights in the interpretation of amplitude/phase patterns in dynamic scintigraphic imaging. Since 1977 we developped in our hospital a TFT as a functional imaging procedure on a dedicated nuclear medicine minicomputer system, (Informatek Simis 4), allowing a generalised application of amplitude/phase analysis in routine clinical use. The first 3 chapters describe the potential applications of a TFT as a functional imaging procedure. The first chapter is based on an intuitive formulation of the concepts of amplitude and phase as parameters for functional imaging. The methodological aspects involved with the use of a TFT as a "general purpose" functional imaging procedure are described. The clinical applicability of these concepts is illustrated with superior vena cavography as an example of a transient phenomenon and with the study of regional breathing patterns by means of dynamic transmission scintigraphy as an example of a periodic phenomenon (Chapters 2 and 3). The rest of the monograph is devoted to data processing of equilibrium gated cardiac blood pool studies. Chapter 4 describes the amplitude and phase images in general as a temporal condensate of an averaged cardiac cycle. The clinical applicability of amplitude phase images for the assessment of regional wall motion disturbances is evaluated in Chapter 5. Chapters 6 and 7 are both clinical studies of patients with coronary artery disease in which the evaluation of regional wall motion is essential. Chapter 8 describes the alterations in amplitude phase patterns resulting from disturbances in electrical activation of the ventricles. From these clinical applications, based on a purely subjective description of amplitude phase images evolved a more fundamental insight into the characteristics of optimisation procedures for the visualisation of activity/time relations in scintigraphic studies (Chapter 9). Finally, Chapter 10 defines indices of cardiac status which quantify structural ventricular disorders in terms of magnitude and timing of motion. This opens new perspectives for the measurement of the efficiency of the heart, describing the ventricles as anisotropic pumps.

REFERENCES

1.  Goris M.L., Thomas A.J., Bell G.B. 1979. Aspects of radionuclide functional imaging of the heart. In : Proc. Intern. Symp. Fundamentals in Technical Progress. Garsou J., Gordenne W., Merchie G. (Eds).
2.  Kaihara S., Natarajan T.K., Wagner Jr H.N. et al. 1969. Construction of a functional image from regional rate constants. J.Nucl.Med. 10, 347.

3. Loken M.K., Medina J.R., Lillehei J.P. 1969. Regional pulmonary function evolution using Xenon-133, a scintillation camera and computer. Radiology 93, 1261.
4. De Roo M.J.K., Goris M., Van Der Schueren G. et al. 1969. Computerized dynamic scintigraphy of the lungs. Respiration 26, 408.
5. Leese J.A., Novak C.S., Taylor V.R. 1970. The determination of cloud pattern motions from geosynchronous satellite image data. Pattern Recognition 2, 279.
6. Di Paola R., Berche C., Bazin J.P. 1974. Traitement digital des information scintigraphiques. In : Proc. 12th Int. Ann. Meeting of the Soc.Nucl.Med., 670.
7. Schmidlin P., Clorius J., Lorenz W.J. 1979. Pattern recognition in renography. In : Information Processing in Medical Imaging - INSERM 88, 335.
8. Oppenheim D., Appeldorn C. 1971. Functional renal imaging using factor analysis. In : Information Processing in Medical Imaging - INSERM 88, 321.
9. Bazin J.P., Di Paola R. 1982. Advances in Factor Analysis Applications in Dynamic Function Studies. In: Nuclear Medicine and Biology - Raynaud C. (Ed.), 35.
10. Cavailloles F., Bazin J.P., Di Paola R., et al., 1982, Factor Analysis in Dynamic Cardiac Studies at Equilibrium. In: Nuclear Medicine and Biology III, Raynaud C. (Ed.), 2361.
11. Britton K.E., Brown N.J.G., Cruz F. et al. 1975. Deconvolution analysis of dynamic studies. In : Information Processing in Scintigraphy. Raynaud C., Todd-Pokropek A. (Eds)., 244.
12. Erbsman F., Ham H., Piepsz A. et al. 1978. Validation of the calculation of the renal impulse response function. An analysis of errors and systematic biases. Biosigma 78 485.
13. Adam W.E., Bitter F. 1981. Advances in heart imaging. In : Medical Radionuclide Imaging. IAEA-SM 247, 195.
14. Schelbert H.R., Verba J.W., Johnson A.D. et al. 1975. Nontraumatic determination of left ventricular ejection fraction by radionuclide angiocardiography. Circulation 51, 902.
15. Geffers H., Meyer G., Bitter F. et al. 1975. Analysis of heart function by gated blood pool investigations (Camera-Kinematography). In : Information Processing in Scintigraphy. Raynaud C., Todd-Pokropek A. (Eds), 462.
16. Geffers H., Adam W.E., Bitter F. et al. 1977. Data processing and functional imaging in radionuclide angiography. In : Proc. 5th Intern. Conf. on Processing in Med. Imaging, 322.
17. Perry J.R., Mosher C.E. 1981. Factors influencing the choice of a nuclear medicine computer system. Clin. Nucl. Med. 6, 19

# 1. THE TEMPORAL FOURIER TRANSFORM AS A GENERAL APPROACH TO FUNCTIONAL ISOTOPIC IMAGING.

## 1.1. AMPLITUDE AND PHASE AS PARAMETERS FOR FUNCTIONAL IMAGING.

Any function $f(t)$ that is periodic with the frequency $\omega = 2\pi/T$ (T = period) can be written mathematically as :

$$
\begin{aligned}
f(t) = \ &A_0 &&\text{0 frequency term - average value}\\
&+ A_1 \cos(\omega t + \phi 1) &&\text{1st harmonic - fundamental frequency}\\
&+ A_2 \cos(2\omega t + \phi 2) &&\text{2nd harmonic}\\
&+ A_3 \cos(3\omega t + \phi 3) &&\text{3rd harmonic}
\end{aligned}
$$

This mathematical procedure which analyses a periodic function into its harmonic components is called Fourier analysis.

Figure 1 illustrates graphically that any periodic function is equal to a sum of simple harmonic functions. These functions are defined by their respective amplitudes $(A_1, A_2, A_3, \ldots)$ and phases $(\phi 1, \phi 2, \phi 3)$.

10

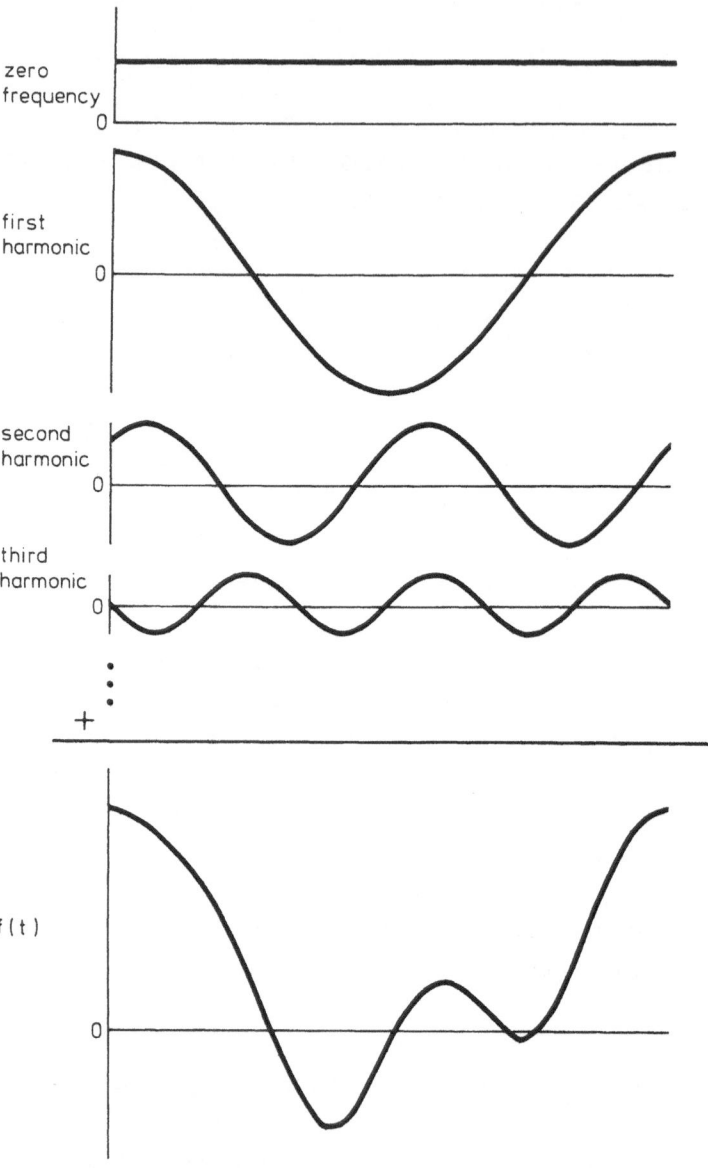

Fig. 1. Graphical representation of Fourier analysis. One period is shown.

Our aim is to discuss the application of a discrete temporal Fourier transform (TFT) on a time series of images, concentrating on the change in the information contained in each pixel as a function of time over the image series (1).

The data present in the image of a dynamic series vary as a discrete function of time (t) and space (x,y). Each pixel in the series is proportional to a number of photons (counts) detected in that particular point (x,y,t) to which the pixel corresponds. In the case of periodic phenomena, the number of counts accumulated in a fixed pixel, varies periodically as a function of time at a frequency equal to the frequency of the periodic phenomenon, such as represented in figure 1. From the mathematical point of view, any function f(t) which is not periodic but defined within an interval (-L,L), such as in transient phenomena, can be made periodic by defining f(t + 2L) = f(t). Fourier analysis can then be applied to this newly defined function. Therefore a time window corresponding to the transient phenomenon has to be choosen (Fig. 2) as this window defines the interval (-L,L).

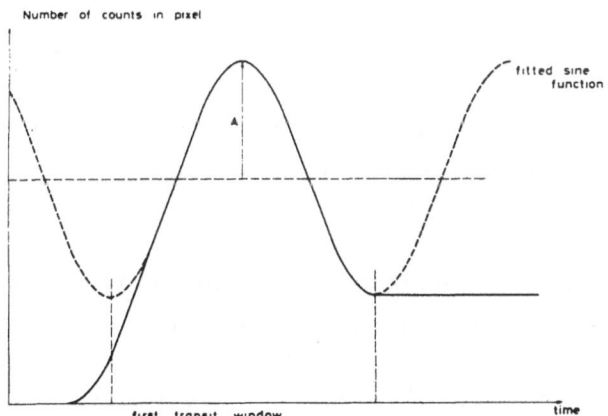

Fig. 2. The transient change in activity approximated by a sine function.

Let I $(x,y,t)$ = $I_1(x,y)$, $I_2(x,y)$,..., $I_i(x,y)$,..., $I_n(x,y)$ be the original image series (periodic or made periodic). The function I $(x,y,t)$ can be written as:

$$I(x,y,t,) = A_0(x,y) \qquad \text{0th harmonic}$$
$$+ \; B_1 \sin \omega t \; + \; C_1 \cos \omega t \qquad \text{1st harmonic}$$
$$+ \; B_2 \sin 2\omega t \; + \; C_2 \cos 2\omega t \qquad \text{2nd harmonic}$$
$$+ \; B_3 \sin 3\omega t \; + \; C_3 \cos 3\omega t \qquad \text{3rd harmonic}$$
$$+ \; ... \qquad\qquad\qquad ...$$

For each pixel $(x,y)$, $A_0$, $B_1$, $C_1$,..., $B_j$, $C_j$,... can be calculated. (to shorten the notation, we delete the brackets $(x,y)$)

$$A_0 = \frac{1}{n} \sum_{i=1}^{n} I_i \; ; \qquad B_j = \frac{2}{n} \sum_{i=1}^{n} I_i \sin \{ j \frac{2\pi}{n} (i-1)\} \; ;$$

$$C_j = \frac{2}{n} \sum_{i=1}^{n} I_j \cos \{ j \frac{2\pi}{n} (i-1)\} \; ; \; ...$$

Introducing the amplitude and the phase yields for each pixel:
$$A = (B^2 + C^2)^{1/2}$$
$$\phi = \text{arctg} \; (-B/C)$$

$$I(t) = A_0 \qquad \text{0th harmonic}$$
$$+ \; A_1 \cos (\omega t + \phi_1) \qquad \text{1th harmonic}$$
$$+ \; A_2 \cos (2\omega t + \phi_2) \qquad \text{2nd harmonic}$$
$$+ \; A_3 \cos (3\omega t + \phi_3) \qquad \text{3rd harmonic}$$
$$+ \; ....$$

The power expansion is exact in the limit where the harmonic $\to \infty$ or, when the function $I(t)$ is limited in frequency, once the highest harmonic present in the function is reached.

In this monograph we will concentrate mostly on the fundamental frequency of the phenomenon. Calculating the first harmonic amplitude and phase for each pixel is equivalent to fitting a sinusoidal function $A \sin (\omega t + \phi)$ to the periodic variation of the number of counts. A is the amplitude of the fitted sine function and $\phi$ is the phase of the same function.

A fit on all (e.g. 4096) pixels of the consecutive images of the dynamic series will yield the two functional parameters for each pixel, the amplitude and the phase respectively. The two parameters are used to yield two functional images. The amplitude image shows the amplitude of the harmonic component of the change in information at the fundamental frequency of each pixel during the periodic cycle. The phase image shows the relative phase of the harmonic component of the change in information, again calculated for each pixel during the whole cycle. By analogy images representing second or higher harmonic amplitudes and phase can also be calculated.

## 1.2. THE CALCULATION OF THE FUNCTIONAL IMAGES

Let $I_1,\ldots, I_i,\ldots, I_n$ be the original image series. Two images, respectively $I_{cos}$ and $I_{sin}$ are calculated :

$$I_{cos} = \sum_{i=1}^{n} I_i \cos \left\{ \frac{2\pi}{n} ( i - 1 )\right\}$$

$$I_{sin} = \sum_{i=1}^{n} I_i \sin \left\{ \frac{2\pi}{n} ( i - 1 )\right\}$$

The amplitude image I AMPL is given by

$$I\ AMPL = (I^2_{cos} + I^2_{sin})^{1/2}$$

The phase image I PHASE is given by

$$I\ PHASE = arctg\ (- I_{sin}/I_{cos})$$

Figure 3 illustrates how both functional images are generated in the case of an equilibrium gated cardiac blood pool study. All images (a) are multiplied with their respective cosine (b) and sine (c) values. Both series are added to form the cosine and sine images (d). From these images, amplitude and phase images are calculated. (All color illustrations are to be found at the back of the book).

## 1.3. SIMULATION STUDIES

### 1.3.1. Periodic phenomenon

A 64 x 64 image matrix was constructed in which each pixel was numbered between 0 and 4095, starting from 0 at the bottom right. Row by row, each pixel was filled with a number of counts equal to the pixel number, giving rise to an image with smoothly increasing intensity from bottom to top (Fig. 4). The image defines the color code used for the amplitude display. In order to simulate a periodic phenomenon, the image was rotated sixteen times around the image center over respective angles of (n x 0.39) radians (n = 0 to 15) to yield sixteen images in which the data rotate once during one complete cycle.

The amplitude image shows the linear increase in amplitude from the center of the image towards the border where the variations in count rate are maximal during the rotatory movement. The color code is shown on the extreme left border of the image. The phase image shows the continuously increasing phase angle represented by a cyclic color code. The phase image defines the color code used for the phase display (cf. 1.4.1.). The corners of the amplitude image show an artifact which is not seen on the phase image. The changes in count rate at the corners of the image are strongly non-harmonic and approach repetitive impulses. A fitted sine function will only reflect the exact amplitude in the case of a pure harmonic function.

## 1.3.2. Non-periodic phenomenon

An image matrix was constructed in which the data was
confined to nine lines, with a normal distribution of the
counts over the columns and a constant distribution over the
rows (Fig. 5). In order to simulate a first pass study, the
image was shifted down over 4 matrix elements fifteen times
to yield sixteen images in which the data roll down once
during the study. The amplitude image shows a constant
amplitude over the image surface. The phase image shows the
increasing phase angle representative for the time of
transit between top and bottom.

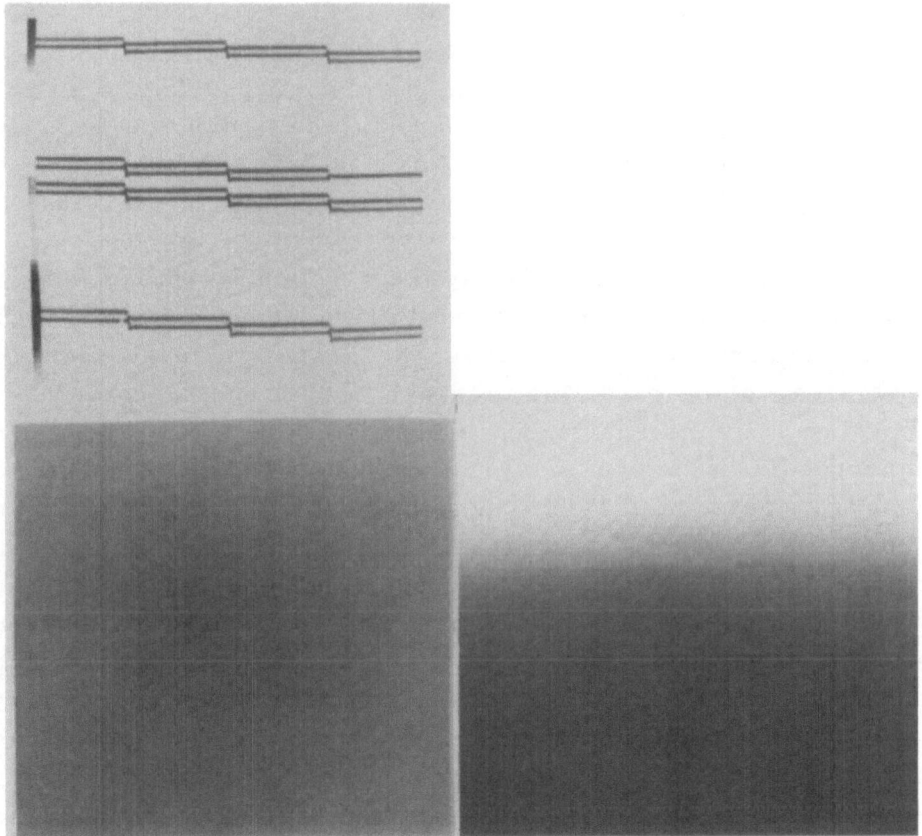

Fig.5. Simulation study of a non periodic phenomenon

## 1.4. DISPLAY OF AMPLITUDE AND PHASE

### 1.4.1. Cyclic color scale

The amplitude can be visualised using an incremental code (color or monochrome). The phase however is a cyclic parameter and the only possible choice for an unequivocal visualisation is a cyclic color code (2). We therefore developed a color code in which each phase angle can be represented by 240 color levels in such a way that the three basic colors of the TV are located at 120 degrees from each other (Fig. 4.c.)

For comparison, figure 6 illustrates how the phase image of the simulation study is represented in different conventional color codes. Note that the cyclic color code associated with the TFT allows a much higher phase resolution than the sampling frequency of the acquisition.

The phase image is displayed as a 64 x 64 image matrix without interpolation. Interpolation is used in digital image restoration to overcome the effect of the discrete spatial sampling rate. The original image can be restored by applying sine interpolation to a finer grid, or by bilinear interpolation. A typical grid is $256^2$. The interpolation assumes continuously changing spatial structures. In functional imaging such a phase imaging, the parameter changes may not be continuous but abrupt, e.g. phase changes between the ventricles and atria. The interpolation between sharp transitions yields smoothly varying values of the parameters that are nor mathematically, nor clinically acceptable. In the particular case of phase imaging, the parameter which is displayed is cyclic with a modulus of 360° or $2\pi$. In the literature, it is common to find phase values in the atria centered around 0° or 360° with pixels of both values situated next to each other. Despite the difference in pixel value (0 or 360), they represent the same phase angle. Interpolating between those pixels introduces pixels with phase values of 180° which, again, are nor mathematically, nor clinically acceptable. We therefore always show the phase images without interpolation.

## 1.4.2. Amplitude modulated phase display

Whenever the amplitude is zero the phase is undefined. In regions with low activity variations, the phase images show large amounts of noise, Therefore it might be useful to combine the phase and amplitude images by modulating the phase image by the amplitude image, i.e. to brighten it differentially in those regions where amplitude excursions are greatest. As the visual perception of colors is strongly function of their intensity, we have not adopted that display technique.

In order to eliminate erroneous phase values induced by noise, all pixels with an amplitude below a given threshold are set black in the phase display (Fig.3e). The threshold value is choosen in function of the statistical noise in the original data series (3).

18

## 1.4.3. Amplitude/phase distribution

The display of the amplitude and phases on a pixel per pixel basis as functional images allows to identify their spatial distribution. A complementary approach consists in calculating the (amplitude weighted) phase distribution function within a particular region of interest (ROI) (3, 4, 5). The phase distribution function is then represented as a histogram using the same color code as for the phase image display (Fig. 3e). Originally, phase distribution histograms were developed as an aid to the comprehension of phase maps displayed in incremental color codes with interpolation (3). However, it is a standard technique in digital image processing to analyse statistically the shape of the first order image histograms as a means of concise image feature extraction (6). Their use in phase maps stimulated the search for describing regional wall motion quantitatively in a standardised manner by the calculation of numerical parameters of the phase distribution in each region (7, 8). The phase distribution can also be displayed in polar coordinates with a cyclic color code rather than in an orthogonal coordinate system (9).

An alternative display represents the amplitude/phase distribution in a complex plane (10). In that approach, each point (x,y) within a ROI is transformed into a point (X,Y) of the complex plane such that

$$X + iY = A_1(x,y) (\cos \phi 1(x,y) + isin \phi 1(x,y))$$

Thus for each point (x,y), the length of its transformed vector corresponds to its amplitude, the angle to the phase angle. The intensity of the X,Y point corresponds to the number of (x,y) pixels with identical amplitude and phase. Instead of the amplitude, the regional ejection fraction can be used as vector length.

## 1.5. DISCUSSION

This chapter was not intended as a comprehensive description of the discrete Fourier transform, but rather as an introduction to the concepts of first harmonic amplitude and phase, as used in functional imaging. For a more comprehensive description of discrete Fourier transforms, the reader is referred to the specialised literature (6, 11, 12).

REFERENCES

1.  Bossuyt A., Deconinck F., Block P. et al. 1979. Improved assessment of regional wall motion disturbances by temporal Fourier transform. (Abstr.) Invest. Radiol. 14, 391.
2.  Deconinck F., Bossuyt A., Hermanne A. 1979. A cyclic color scale as an essential requirement in functional imaging of periodic phenomena. Med. Phys. 6, 331.
3.  Bitter F., Adam W.E., Geffers H. et al. 1979. Synchronised steady state heart investigation. In : Intern. Symp. Fundamentals in Technical Progress. Vol.III, 9.1.
4.  Links J.M., Douglas H.K., Wagner H.N. 1980. Patterns of ventricular emptying by Fourier analysis of gated blood pool studies. J.Nucl.Med. 21, 978.
5.  Pavel D., Byrom E., Swiryn S. et al. 1980. Normal and abnormal electrical activation of the heart : imaging patterns obtained by phase analysis of equilibrium cardiac studies. Medical Radionuclide Imaging II - IAEA-SM 247, 253.
6.  Pratt W.K. 1978. Digital Image processing. Wiley Interscience Publication.
7.  Byrom E., Pavel D.G., Meyer-Pavel C. 1981. Phase images of gated cardiac studies: A standard evaluation procedure. In: Functional Mapping of Organ Systems. Esser P.(Ed.) 129.
8.  Bacharach S., Green M., Bonow R. et al. 1982. A method for objective evaluation of functional images. J. Nucl. Med. 23, 285.
9.  Adam W.E. 1982. Cardiac Function. In: Nuclear Medicine and Biology II Raynaud C. (Ed.) 2149.
10. Liehn J.C., Valeyre J., Collet E. et al. 1981. Etude de la cinétique ventriculaire régionale par représentation dans le plan complexe. Proc. XXIIe Coll. de Méd. Nucl. de Langue Fran., 55.
11. Huang T.S. 1981. Two-dimensional Digital Signal Processing I In: Topics in Applied Physics Vol 42.
12. Castleman K.R. 1979. The Fourier Transform In: Digital Image Processing Castleman K.R. (Ed.) 161.

# 2. AMPLITUDE / PHASE IMAGING OF TRANSIENT PHENOMENA: SUPERIOR CAVOGRAPHY.

## 2.1. INTRODUCTION

Many nuclear medicine procedures study the impulse/response of an anatomical structure to the administration of a radioactive tracer localised in time. The most straightforward example is probably radioisotope angiography. Whenever a radiotracer is injected intravenously the first transit through an organ can be followed in order to estimate the regional blood flow. The technical requirements are: a bolus injection of the tracer and the acquisition of a dynamic series of images with sufficient time resolution. The most important limitation of first pass studies is the poor signal to noise ratio in the individual images. Quantification is therefore generally reduced to the calculation of time/activity curves within a region of interest. In that way most of the spatial information is lost.

Parametric functional images of first transit regional blood flow studies calculate for each pixel the maximum (max) and the maximum appearance time (tmax) during the time interval of the first passage of the tracer (1). These images are strongly dependent on statistical noise. We therefore compared amplitude and phase images with conventional max or tmax images for superior vena caval imaging. Isotopic cavography was used to study mediastinal flow obstruction induced by retrosternal goiters.

Although rare, a benign superior vena cava syndrome can have numerous etiologies, substernal goiter being one of them (2). In this study we describe 5 patients, 3 of them with substernal goiter associated with a superior vena cava syndrome. In 2 of them, the syndrome presented an intermittent waxing and waning pattern. We suspected the degree of neck flexion to be responsible for the position of the substernal goiter relative to the great veins in the mediastinum: neck flexion could result in further descent of the substernal goiter and thereby enhance venous compression. To test this hypothesis, radionuclide superior cavography was performed first with the neck in extension and repeated with the neck in flexion. The results of these 3 patients were compared to those obtained in 2 patients with substernal goiter without clinically apparent superior vena cava obstruction and in 5 control subjects.

## 2.2. DATA ACQUISITION AND PROCESSING

Radionuclide superior cavography was performed with the patient immobilised in supine position the arms spread apart. A large field of view gamma camera was positioned anteriorly above the upper thorax and neck. After 5 minutes of immobilisation in this position to allow cardiac output to return to steady state resting values, equal doses (1.5 to 2 mCi in 1 ml volume) of $^{99m}$Tc pertechnetate were injected simultaneously as bolusses into symmetric veins of each arm, with the neck of the patient in extension. One hundred 0.5 sec digitised images were obtained. During the whole procedure normal tidal breathing was asked for, to avoid alterations in blood flow induced by Valsalva manoeuver. Thereafter, the whole procedure was repeated as described above, with the subject's neck 45 degrees flexed by positioning a pad under his head.

From the original images a series of 24 successive images was selected starting with the first image on which both bolusses were visualised in the gamma camera field of view. After preprocessing by a 9 point spatial smoothing and a time smoothing with kernel (1,2,1), the image series was used for the calculation of max, tmax, first harmonic amplitude and phase functional images. From the images obtained, we analysed the flow pattern of the tracer, the presence or absence of collateral circulation, the site of venous obstruction and the transit time (TT), defined here as the duration of tracer passage from the subclavian veins to the right atrium, in whatever way this occured.

The study group consisted of 5 patients with substernal goiter; of these 3 presented with a the superior vena cava syndrome (cases 1,2 and 3), while the other 2 patients presented with an asymptomatic superior mediastinal mass, detected on chest radiography, without signs or symptoms of superior vena cava obstruction (cases 4 and 5). The control group consisted of 5 subjects without thyroid disease or superior vena cava syndrome, and normal mediastinum on chest roentgenogram.

2.3. RESULTS

Figure 7.a shows the preprocessed series of images representing the first transit of the tracer through the mediastinum in a normal control subject. Figure 7.b represents the max, tmax, amplitude and phase images. The functional images allow a better distinction of the different anatomical structures than is possible by a visual inspection of the time series alone. The information content of the max and the amplitude image and of the tmax and the phase image is similar. The calculation of first harmonic amplitude and phase however is less influenced by the signal to noise ratio present in the original data. This is illustrated in Figure 7.c in which the same functional images were calculated on the image series without preprocessing.

In all 5 control subjects free passage of the tracer through the normal venous pathways was observed bilaterally, and flow occured simultaneously on both sides, both with neck in extension and in flexion. With neck extension TT ranged from 2.5 to 4.5 s for the 5 control subjects, with neck flexion TT ranged from 2 to 3.5 s. (Table 1).

Table 1. Transit time measurements in control group.

|     | Age | Sex | TT(sec) ext. | flex. |
| --- | --- | --- | --- | --- |
| SO  | 28  | M   | 3.5 | 3.5 |
| RO  | 28  | M   | 4.5 | 3.5 |
| VI  | 29  | M   | 3.5 | 3.0 |
| ST  | 19  | F   | 2.5 | 2.0 |
| LA  | 61  | M   | 3.5 | 3.0 |

Legend : M = male ; F = Female ; ext. = neck extension ; flex. = neck flexion.

In the five patients with substernal goiter TTs were significantly prolonged with neck extension as compared to the normals. Since no systematic differences were observed in flow pattern or TT between patients with and without superior vena cava syndrome, their results are considered together in table 2. With neck extension TT ranged from 3.5 to 9 s, 2 patients had a TT within the normal range because venous flow was unimpeded on one of the two sides. With neck flexion, the TT was prolonged in all 5 patients and reached a value well above the normal range (5.5 to 16 s).

Table 2. Transit time measurements in patients with substernal goiter.

|  | Age | Sex | SVC syndrome | TT (sec) ext. | TT (sec) flex. | after surgery TT (sec) ext. | after surgery TT (sec) flex. |
|---|---|---|---|---|---|---|---|
| MA | 68 | M | intermittent | 6.0 | 16.0 | 5.5 | 6.0 |
| VA | 69 | M | fixed | 4.0 | 7.0 | 2.5 | 2.5 |
| GE | 70 | F | intermittent | 9.0 | 10.0 | - | - |
| HE | 65 | F | - | 9.0 | 12.0 | - | - |
| MO | 62 | F | - | 3.5 | 5.5 | - | - |

Legend : M = male ; F = female ; ext. = neck extension ; flex. = neck flexion.

Figure 8 represents the functional images obtained in patient 1. With neck extension normal tracer passage occured from the left side, while it was very slow from the right side. No collaterals were visible. With neck flexion, tracer passage was delayed on the left side and completely obstructed on the right side at the level of the innominate vein. These findings were confirmed by radiographic contrast cavography. One month after surgical removal of a large colloidal goiter of 220 grams, the flow pattern and TT were returned to normal, without any influence from the position of the neck.

In patient 2, passage of the tracer was abolished through normal channels with neck flexion, whereas passage preferentially took place bilaterally via collaterals (fig. 9). With neck extension TT was prolonged and the tracer passed bilaterally through both normal and collateral channels. One month after excision of a large colloidal goiter (192 grams), collaterals were no longer visible but TT was still prolonged with neck extension. However TT did not significantly increase with neck flexion.

In patient 3 tracer passage occured predominantly on the left side with neck extension but was very slow. With neck flexion, the TT was slightly longer and the right innominate vein was now completely occluded as shown by stagnation of the tracer in the right subclavian vein. No collaterals were visible in either position. In patient 4 with neck extension, tracer passage occured slowly through normal and collateral channels. With neck flexion, the tracer passed only through collateral channels. In patient 5 TT and flow pattern were normal with neck extension. However, with neck flexion, flow was occluded at the level of the right innominate vein and substantially slowed on the left side. No collaterals were visible.

## 2.4. DISCUSSION

The superior vena cava is the ideal vessel for isotope angiography. Any upper extremity injection will drain into the superior vena cava without significant attenuation of the bolus and there is sufficient time between the first appearance of activity and the loss of definition secondary to the pulmonary capillary bed. Radionuclide superior cavography is a simple, noninvasive and repeatable procedure for initial screening and follow up studies of the superior vena cava syndrome, especially when mediastinal invasion of a neoplasm is suspected (3,4).

As shown by our patients radionuclide superior cavography can demonstrate subclinically present or impending venous obstruction. From the results we obtained, it is clear that the position of the neck is an important factor for the diagnostic accuracy of the test. These findings strongly suggest that neck posture directly influences the position of a substernal goiter, or any mass situated at the thoracic inlet, relative to the mediastinal vessels, provided the mass is not fixed and can be mobilised. With neck flexion, such a mass descends further down into the superior mediastinum and the there situated compliant vessels undergo further compression or even complete occlusion. When the neck is extended, the mobile mass is elevated, compression relieved and venous flow facilitated. An unexpected finding from this study was that there was no difference on radionuclide superior cavography between the goiter patients with and without superior vena cava syndrome. In the presence of superior mediastinal masses, venous flow abnormalities in the superior vena cava system might be more common than previously thought.

As the impulse response can easily be defined in the case of radionuclide superior cavography, the characteristics of the functional imaging procedure can be recognised: the information in time and space of the image series is compressed into 2 images. The first image represents the distribution in space of the importance of the response, the second image the timing of the response. Maximum and time of maximum are in this respect the most straightforward parameters. Their determination makes no assumption about a mathematical formulation of the impulse response. Amplitude and phase images assume a model for the temporal behaviour of the changes in activity of each pixel over the image series. The approximation by a sinusoidal function is rather crude and has no physiological counterpart. Nevertheless, as the information density contained in the whole image series is considered rather than the density of each individual image, the statistical value of the study is markedly improved (5,6). The first harmonic functional images correspond to an extreme low frequency filter.

Similar bolus progression images have been described by Goris (7). He used the time information of a first transit study in heart and lungs for the automated detection and determination of left to right shunting and for the non-interactive identification of the left ventricular area (8). For studies such as first transit cerebral blood flow or renal blood flow, the approximation of the tracer passage by a sinusoidal function is limited by the change in bolus shape as it passes through various capillary beds. Even then the amplitude/phase display allows a more accurate selection of regions of interest for subsequent analysis.

REFERENCES

1.  Budinger T.F., De Land F.H., Duggan H.E. et al. 1975.
    Dynamic time-dependant analysis and static three-
    dimensional imaging procedures for computer assisted CNS
    studies. In : Non Invasive Brain Imaging. De Blanc H.J.,
    Sorensen J.A. (Eds), 45.
2.  Mahajan V., Strimlan V., Van Ordstrand H.S., Loop F.D.
    1975. Benign superior vena cava syndrome. Chest 69, 32.
3.  Maxfield W.S., Meckstroth G.R. 1969. Tc-99m superior
    vena cavography. Radiology 92, 913.
4.  Van Houte P., Fruhling J. Radionuclide venography in the
    evaluation of superior vena cava syndrome. 1981. Clin.
    Nucl. Med. 6, 177.
5.  Bossuyt A., Deconinck F., Lepoudre R. et al. 1979 The
    temporal Fourier Transform applied to functional
    isotopic imaging. INSERM 88, 397.
6.  Deconinck F., Bossuyt A., Jonckheer M. et al. 1979.
    Functional imaging in first pass isotopic angiography.
    Eur.J. Nucl. Med. 4, 132.
7.  Goris M.L., Wallington J., Baum D. et al. 1976. Nuclear
    angiography automated selection of regions of interest
    for the generation of time activity curves and
    parametric image display and interpretation. Clin. Nucl.
    Med. 1, 99.
8.  Goris M.L. 1978. Non-interactive identification of the
    left ventricular area. In : Nuclear Cardiology :
    Selected Computer Aspects. Sorensen J.A. (Ed.), 139.

# 3. REGIONAL BREATHING PATTERNS STUDIED BY DYNAMIC TRANSMISSION SCINTIGRAPHY AND THE TEMPORAL FOURIER TRANSFORM

## 3.1. INTRODUCTION

Standard lung ventilation or perfusion scintigraphy does not take into account the movement and the expansion of the lungs during respiration. Attempts to take these factors into account using dynamic lung imaging aimed at improving the static image quality by correcting the images for the changes which occur during respiration (1). It was our aim to take advantage of the information contained in a dynamic series of lung images by studying the breathing mechanism rather than correcting for it.

In this study we describe the use of amplitude/phase functional images obtained by Temporal Fourier Transform (TFT) to evaluate the possibility of detecting differences in mechanical behaviour of the lungs induced by different breathing manoeuvres in healthy individuals or induced by disease in COPD patients (2).

## 3.2. DETECTION METHOD

Density changes in the lungs during the respiratory cycle can be expressed in terms of changes in x- or gamma ray transmission, reflecting the local air/tissue (and blood) volume ratio. These changes in transmission depend on:
a)  local changes in lung expansion in a plane perpendicular to the direction of the transmission beam,
b)  organ displacement as a result of respiratory movements (e.g. subdiaphragmatic abdominal organs),
c)  local variations in blood volume due to vascular pulsations (3).

We previously described a modified transmission densitometry technique using a $^{99m}$Tc point source and a large field of view gamma camera without collimator, in a classical radiological disposition (4). The classical roentgenfilm with its high spatial resolution is replaced in this technique by a time sensitive single photon detector. In order to analyse such dynamic density changes, long exposure times are needed. The limited spatial resolution of the detector is of minor importance due to the motion blurring during respiration and due to the limited number of photons in each image. This disposition allows the regional visualisation of dynamic changes in gamma ray transmission through the thorax during the respiratory cycle, with negligible radiation burden for the patient (5).

Earlier scintigraphic transmission studies used a gamma camera collimator system as such and a flood field $^{99m}$Tc source in front of the patient (6,7). It is well known that the best spatial resolution of gamma cameras is obtained by accumulating a transmission image of a 100% contrast phantom (Bar, Anger, ...) on a gamma camera without collimator, using an isotopic point source far enough from the camera crystal plane in order to obtain a homogeneous radiation field. Indeed, the spatial resolution of a gamma camera collimator system is represented by:

$$RS = (Ri + Rc)^{1/2}$$

where Ri is the intrinsic gamma camera resolution and Rc the extrinsic detector or collimator resolution. Deleting the collimator will therefore improve the system resolution. Our recording procedure therefore is as follows: a point source of 5-10 mCi $^{99m}$Tc is placed at 2m from the crystal plane of the detector without collimator, thus being used at maximal sensitivity and intrinsic resolution; in this way the maximal count rate of the gamma camera can be fully utilised. The patient is positioned next to the camera (Fig. 10). The detector system is interfaced to a data storage and processing system.

TRANSMISSION SCINTIGRAPHY :

* Tc-99m   POINT SOURCE ( 5 mCi )
  2m FROM CAMERA ( NO COLLIMATOR )

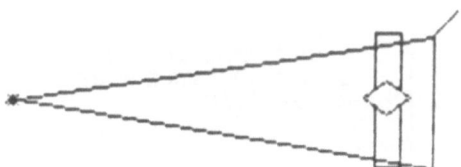

Fig.10. Recording procedure of transmission images.

Dynamic acquisition of a number of respiratory cycles
was obtained by recording 140 images of 0.5 sec.,
respectively 0.2 sec., during slow (yielding 12 respiratory
cycles of 20 images) and fast (resulting in 24 respiratory
cycles of 10 images) breathing rates. In this aspect the
detection technique is different from most other digital
radiography techniques that use high incident photon fluxes.
Here the photon flux is so low, that single photon counting
is performed.

## 3.3. DATA PROCESSING

A series of similar cycles was reduced into one average
respiratory cycle by adding the different cycles taking the
image representing maximal inspiration (TLC) as the starting
point of each cycle. This image can be recognised because it
contains maximal count rates (Fig. 11). Atypical cycles,
which were either too short or too long were omitted.

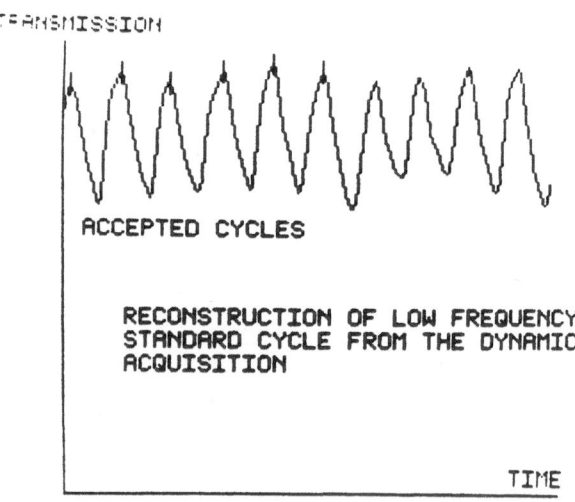

Fig. 11. Selection of cycle length for the reconstruction of
an averaged respiratory cycle.

The thus obtained averaged cycles consisted of 10 to 20 images. Each of these averaged respiratory cycles were representative of the series which they averaged and were analysed by generating time/activity curves over top and bases of the lungs. A TFT was applied to each of these average representative cycles. Both parameters were represented as functional images by use of an appropriate color code to study amplitude and phase of the phenomenon at its fundamental frequency and in the form of a phase distribution histogram modulated by the amplitude. Figure 12 illustrates a processed data series obtained during erect FB.

## 3.4. BREATHING PATTERNS IN HEALTHY INDIVIDUALS

The influence of respiratory rate, body posture and breathing pattern on the cyclic variations in gamma ray transmission of different lung regions was studied in 4 young healthy non-smoking individuals. Three breathing patterns were studied: fast breathing (FB: 30 cycles/min), slow breathing (6 cycles/min), using preferentially the abdominal (SAB) or the thoracic/intercostal (STB) musculature. Each of these three breathing patterns, FB, SAB and STB, was carried out in 2 different body postures: standing erect and supine. Postero-anterior and lateral views were recorded on each of these six breathing manoeuvres.

The greatest amplitudes of the changes in transmission are situated at the lung basis in both erect and supine postures reflecting transmission changes due to rostro-caudal displacement of the diaphragm and abdominal contents. Since in all three breathing manoeuvres near inspiratory capacity breaths were taken, the resulting diaphragm excursions are nearly equal. Another zone of high

amplitudes, more apparent during slow thoracic and fast
breathing patterns and best seen on the lateral views is the
retrosternal zone due to dorsoventral displacement of the
thoracic cage (Fig. 13). Although these changes in amplitude
reflect thoracic cage and diaphragmatic movements, they
clearly directly influence the expansion of the immediately
underlying lung zones (chest wall-lung interdependence). The
amplitude changes of the FB pattern resemble those of the
STB pattern suggesting intercostal/accessory muscle
recruitment during more extreme dynamic breathing conditions
(8).

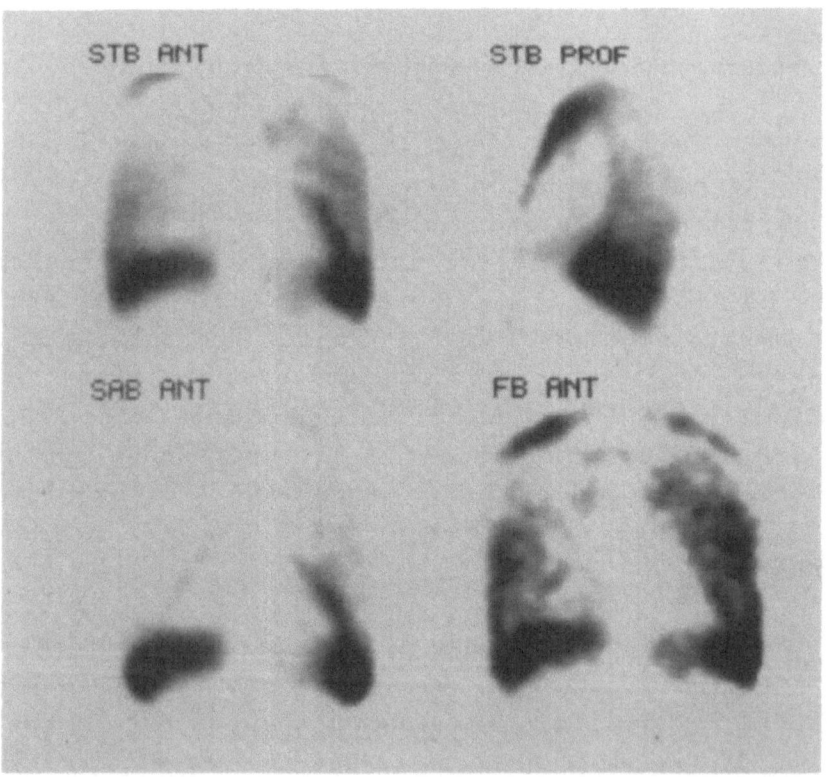

Fig. 13.  Amplitude images obtained with different breathing
manoeuvres.

Table 1 summarizes the effect of the different breathing patterns observed on the synchronicity of transmission changes. During STB, inspiration starts at the apexes while expiration begins at the bases of the lungs. During SAB expiration still begins at the bases but inspiration occurs simultaneously at top and bases. During FB inspiration and expiration of the apexes preceed that of the bases (Fig. 14).

Table 1. Effect of breathing patterns on the synchronicity of transmission changes.

|  | SAB | STB | FB |
|---|---|---|---|
| Inspiration | T = B | T → B | T → B |
| Expiration | T ← B | T ← B | T → B |

T → B : top before base
T = B : top and base simultaneously
T ← B : top after base

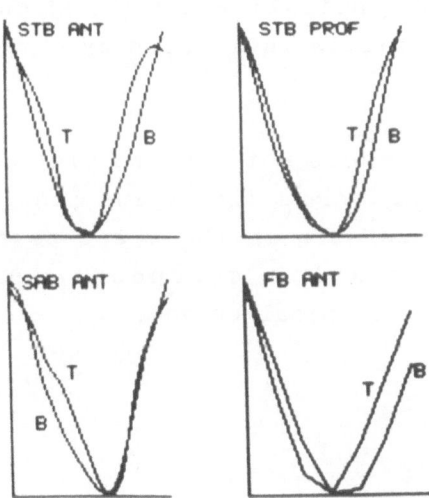

Fig. 14. Time/activity curves over top and bases of the lungs during different breathing manoeuvres.

Phase shifts in young healthy erect adults are minimal during STB (Fig. 15.a and 15.b). They become more evident in the SAB pattern, the lung bases expiring before the apices. Otherwise stated, during STB the phase of lung expansion is fairly uniform, while the SAB pattern provokes phase shifts between basal and apical lung zones. During FB, phase shifts are markedly accentuated as shown by wider amplitude modulated phase histograms and clearly indicate that apical (retrosternal) zones now breath before basal (diaphragmatic) zones.

The amplitude modulated phase histograms indicate that in normal subjects regional asynchronism is almost absent under moderate dynamic breathing conditions. However, under extreme dynamic breathing conditions, when inspiratory flow rates and frequencies are increased, slight asynchronism occurs. This indicates that regional differences in time constants (product of resistance R and compliance C) become important under more extreme dynamic breathing conditions (9). From the phase images, it can be seen that the temporal nonuniformity of ventilation has a regional-topographical basis and that this is influenced by the pattern of muscle contraction.

Body posture does not seem to play an important role, except during SAB, where the supine posture diminishes the phase differences seen in the erect posture, probably by reducing the gravity dependent influence of the subdiaphragmatic abdominal organs.

3.5.  BREATHING PATTERNS IN COPD PATIENTS. EFFECT OF
ABDOMINAL/DIAPHRAGMATIC BREATHING RETRAINING ON
DIAPHRAGMATIC FUNCTION.

Comprehensive management of patients with chronic
obstructive pulmonary disease (COPD) includes physical
therapy consisting of sputum removal by postural drainage
and chest/ percussion/ vibration and breathing retraining.
In COPD patients, as a result of hyperinflation, the
diaphragm, which is normally the main respiratory muscle,
functions poorly (10). Therefore COPD patients excessively
use their accessory and intercostal inspiratory muscles,
which are less efficient pressure generators. Since
augmented abdominal breathing techniques (AAB) promote
greater use of the diaphragm and reduce the use of
intercostal accessory muscles, it is conceivable that AAB
may render breathing more efficient and may improve the
distribution of ventilation. The benefit of breathing
retraining, however, is still controversial, generally being
based on subjective grounds due to the lack of unanimous
objective evidence of improved lung function.

3.5.1. Study protocol

This study concerns 7 COPD patients admitted during
acute exacerbation of their chronic respiratory
insufficiency in which we used the transmission
scintigraphic technique to evaluate the effect of AAB on
their breathing patterns. All patients were studied on two
occasions:
1. during the subacute stage, i.e. a few days after hospital
admission for exacerbation of respiratory failure. At the
time of this study, patients were fairly stable due to
pharmacological therapy, and expiratory flow rates had
returned to baseline values. During data acquisition, the
breathing pattern was "natural" except that breathing

frequency and tidal volume were constant and guided by a physiotherapist.

2. Two to three weeks later, during which period the patients had been instructed in the AAB technique several times daily. AAB consisted of slow, deep inspirations and prolonged expirations against pursed lips. Inspiration was accomplished by preferential diaphragmatic contraction as indicated by enhanced outward movement of the abdominal wall. Towards the end of expiration, active abdominal muscle contraction assisted lung deflation with the aim to reduce FRC. During data acquisition, the patient was breathing at the same frequency and tidal volume as during the first study, but using the AAB technique. This was done in the presence of the physiotherapist who had been treating the patient and who presently coached his breathing. Data acquisition in the seated position, and data processing were performed as previously described.

3.5.2. Results

During the subacute study before AAB training, the amplitude image is more heterogeneous in all 7 COPD patients as compared to normals (Fig.16). In 5 of them, dependent lung regions however still reveal larger amplitudes, and after AAB training they even become more prominent in 2 of these 5 patients. In the 2 patients with the most severe airflow obstruction, the vertical amplitude gradient not only is abolished, but even inverted, the apical nondependent lung regions showing the largest amplitudes. In these 2 patients, AAB retraining markedly increased the amplitude in the dependent lung regions, reverting the image towards a more normal appearance. Therefore in 4 of the 7 patients, AAB retraining was capable of enhancing diaphragmatic excursion and subsequent dependent lung zone ventilation.

Like the amplitude image, the functional phase image is also more heterogeneous in COPD patients as compared to normals, indicating asynchronous behaviour of the different lung regions even during tidal breathing, as a result of interregional time-constant differences. Furthermore in 5 of the 7 patients, large markedly out-of-phase regions can be detected. These regions show good gamma ray transmission and small amplitudes, and correspond to hyperlucent avascular lung zones on chest X-ray in 3 of them. The 2 patients not showing these grossly out-of-phase regions, had unremarkable chest X-rays and reversible airflow limitation on pulmonary function testing. Asynchronous ventilation is exemplified by wider phase/amplitude histograms with larger surface areas in all COPD patients as compared to normal. In 3 of the 7 patients these histograms furthermore had a bimodal appearance. After AAB retraining, phase shifts are reduced in all 7 patients as indicated by a 29% reduction of the histogram surface area (Table 2).

Table 2. Phase/amplitude histogram surface area (in arbitrary units).

| Patient | Before AAB | After AAB | Change in % |
|---------|-----------|-----------|-------------|
| SCH  | 7126  | 7072 | - 0.8  |
| WOU  | 5791  | 4714 | - 18.6 |
| MAT  | 11778 | 7553 | - 35.9 |
| MAC  | 18434 | 9910 | - 46.2 |
| DOQ  | 12437 | 7616 | - 38.7 |
| MIC  | 4849  | 4440 | - 8.4  |
| VAN  | 9210  | 8116 | - 11.9 |
| Mean | 9947  | 7060 | - 29.0 |

### 3.5.3. Comments

The functional amplitude and phase images of COPD patients can easily be distinguished from normal subjects, by their more heterogeneous distribution. Large regions, characterized by high transmission, low amplitude and large phase shifts probably represent emphysematous bullous areas. Using the transmission technique,combined with digital image processing, we provided some evidence of improved diaphragmatic function after AAB retraining. The small number of patients studied does not allow us to separate those patients who will respond to therapy from those who will not. However,the 2 patients with the most heterogeneous pretreatment amplitude image and abolished/reversed amplitude gradient showed the largest changes after AAB retraining. Although we fully realize that most patients do not maintain this learned breathing pattern unconsciously, we believe that it provides them with a more efficient breathing pattern which they can use - and some patients do- when they need it most, i.e. when the respiratory system is stressed during intercurrent bronchial infections or during exercise.

## 3.6. DISCUSSION

The technique which is described is a combination of a digital radiological technique and nuclear medicine image processing (11). As compared to conventional X-ray images, our data are recorded as digital images representing at each point of the image the photon density detected by the gamma camera crystal. By using the NaI detector as a photoncounter and not at saturation (as in CT and other digital radiology techniques), the radiation burden is significantly reduced. The limited spatial resolution or size of the digital detectors which are nowadays available represents a limitation to their use in transmission densitometry techniques.

The dynamic data available by means of the detection method reflect the mechanical effects of breathing. The application of functional imaging procedures to these data allowed to differentiate different breathing patterns in normal individuals, to differentiate normal from pathological states, and to objectivate the effect of therapy in patients. The study therefore illustrates that even crude digital transmission signals from the point of view of spatial resolution may yield dynamic information of physiological and clinical interest. With the future advent of higher quality detectors, information which is nowadays lost in clinical radiological examinations, will become easily accessible.

REFERENCES

1.  Touya J.J., Jones J.P., Price R.R. et al. 1981. Imaging
    of ventilation/perfusion ratio by gated regional
    spirometry. Medical Radionuclide Imaging II - IAEA-SM-
    247, 455.
2.  Bossuyt A., Vincken W., Deconinck F. 1981. Patterns of
    regional lung expansion studied by dynamic tranmission
    scintigraphy and the temporal Fourier transform. In :
    Functional mapping of organ systems and other computer
    topics. Esser (Ed), 57.
3.  Laws J.W., Steiner R.E. 1965. X-ray densitometry in the
    study of pulmonary ventilation and the pulmonary
    circulation. 512.
4.  Deconinck F., Bossuyt A., Lepoudre R. et al. 1979.
    Computerised transmission densitography and tomography
    with a gamma camera. INSERM 88, 245.
5.  Deconinck F. 1978. Transmission densitometry. A modified
    method. J.Belge Radiol. 61, 513.
6.  Kuhl D.E., Hale J., Eaton W.L. 1965. Transmission
    scanning : a useful adjunct to conventional emission
    scanning for accurately keying isotope deposition to
    radiographic anatomy. Radiology 87, 278.
7.  Potchen E.J. et al. 1970. Regional pulmonary function in
    man. Quantitative transmission radiography as an
    adjunct to lung scintiscanning. Radiology 108, 724.
8.  Macklem P.T., Roussos C., Dubois F. et al. 1977.
    Contribution of intercostal and/or accessory inspiratory
    muscles to voluntary increases in inspiratory flow rate.
    Proc. Intern. Union Physiol. Sci. 13, 463.
9.  Otis A.B., McKerrow C.M., Bartlett R.A. et al. 1956.
    Mechanical factors for the distribution of pulmonary
    ventilation. J. Appl. Physiol. 8, 427.
10. Sharp J.T., Danon J., Druz W.S. et al. 1974. Respiratory
    muscle function in patients with chronic obstructive
    pulmonary disease: its relationship to disability and to
    respiratory therapy. Am. Rev. Resp. Dis. 110, 154.
11. Deconinck F., Bossuyt A., Vincken W. et al. 1981.
    Temporal processing of digital radiographs of the
    breathing lung. SPIE - Digital Radiography 314, 110.

# 4. AMPLITUDE/PHASE IMAGES AS A TEMPORAL CONDENSATE OF THE AVERAGED CARDIAC CYCLE

## 4.1. INTRODUCTION

Equilibrium gated nuclear angiocardiography (EGNA) is used to study non invasively the function of the heart considered as a blood pump. EGNA is based on the fact that the heart contracts periodically. A small amount of radioactive tracer which distributes itself into the blood pool is administered to the patient (e.g. 20mCi of $^{99m}$Tc labelled red blood cells). Provided there is a homogeneous mixture of the radioactive tracer in the blood pool, the precordial count rates reflect the cyclic volume changes in the heart. During each R-R interval, a number (e.g. 16) of images of the heart is acquired using a gamma camera. Because the count rate is too low for a single beat-to-beat analysis, imaging is performed using an ECG gating technique in which the images corresponding to a number of individual cycles are added, until the statistical validity of the study is satisfactory (1,2,3,4,5). In a typical EGNA, the amount of data present in the image series is of the order of 65 kbyte. The information content in the dynamic image series is very high, but all the information present in the series is not relevant (e.g. photon noise).

Among the relevant information present in the dynamic image series are temporal patterns which describe the hemodynamic changes. One subjective, but widespread approach to the study of temporal contraction or relaxation patterns is visual inspection of the image series displayed as a movie. The mathematical approaches to study these patterns involve modelisation. One approach assumes a model for the spatial behaviour of the temporal changes in activity and is based on the choice of regions of interest (ROI) in the image. Time/activity curves are generated and global parameters (e.g. left ventricular ejection fraction, ejection rate, maximal rate of left ventricular filling), are extracted from the curve. Within the ROI, all information on spatial variations in temporal behaviour is lost. In this context, it is also possible to use a non imaging detector which can directly produce a left ventricular time/activity curve (when properly collimated and positioned over the left ventricle)(6,7). The second approach assumes a model for the temporal behaviour of the changes in activity in each pixel over the series of images and associates a number of parameters with this behaviour (8). These parameters are then displayed as parametric images. An example is first harmonic Fourier imaging in which each pixel shows the first harmonic phase or amplitude of the pixel time/activity curve (9,10). All information on higher harmonics in the curve is discarded. Functional phase and amplitude imaging overcomes some of the limitations due to individual image noise and to the limited temporal sampling frequency during the digital acquisition.

## 4.2. DATA ACQUISITION

Red cells were labelled in vivo by an i.v. injection of 20 mCi of $^{99m}$Tc pertechnetate preceeded by 3 ng of stannous pyrophosphate (11). After equilibration of the tracer, cardiac blood pool imaging was performed in a modified 45. LAO position to isolate optimally the left ventricle. By use of a gamma camera interfaced to an Informatek Simis 3 processing system, ECG gated data were collected and concurrently organised on a high phase resolution basis (12) into a series of 16 images of 64 x 64 pixels that span an averaged cardiac cycle. Cycles following cycles falling outside a physician selected temporal beat length window were rejected during the data acquisition to prevent distortion of time/activity curves. Preprocessing on the acquired series involved equalisation of the total activity in each image in order to correct gating artefacts, followed by a 9 point spatial and a 3 point temporal smoothing.

## 4.3. INTERPRETATION OF AMPLITUDE AND PHASE IN TERMS OF CARDIAC FUNCTION

The study in figure 17 shows the original 16 images which represent one averaged cardiac cycle obtained from an EGNA study in a normal control person. Image intensity is assumed to be proportional to blood volume. All but the major volume changes (e.g. left ventricle) are invisible because of the superposition of a high stationary structured background. Figure 17.b. represent the end diastolic and the end systolic frames. In these frames, the color of each pixel represents the activity detected in each matrix element. The color code is represented on the left. Three ROI are drawn on the image. They are used to calculate the changes in count rate that occur in the left ventricle (ROI

1), right atrium (ROI 2) and liver (ROI 3) during the averaged cardiac cycle. The time/activity curves calculated for each of the three ROI describe the temporal behaviour of each of these structures as a whole.

First harmonic amplitude/phase analysis is shown in figure 17.c. As in the amplitude image, the color of each pixel corresponds to the amount of changes in count rate that is synchronous with the heart cycle, all stationary background structures such as the liver are completely eliminated from the image. The amplitude image visualises the importance of the volume changes in all heart cavities whenever they occur during the cardiac cycle. As such, the image corresponds to a "stroke volume" image for all heart chambers, which are clearly delineated. The ROI are drawn on the image.

In the phase image, the color of each pixel corresponds to the sequence of the volume changes in ventricles and atria in relation to one another. As expected, there is a phase shift of 180° between ventricles and atria. Where the amplitude is below a choosen threshold, the phase is not determined. The cyclic color code which is used for the phase representation is shown around the image.

The amplitude/phase distribution over the whole heart region has two peaks in normal persons corresponding to the atrial and the ventricular pixels. Within statistical limits, there is no phase shift between right and left ventricle. In normal control persons, the shape and spread of the left ventricular amplitude/phase distribution is tight (s.d.: 12°).

4.4. CINEMATIC DISPLAY OF THE WAVE OF EMPTYING

The use of a cinematic display of the propagation of the wave of emptying was introduced by Verba (13). To determine the point in the cardiac cycle at which the emptying started in each pixel, he used the second derivate of a Fourier filtered time/activity curve. The same kind of information is readily available from the first harmonic phase matrix (14), provided the regional phase differences within the ventricles represent regional differences in systole.

A series of frames can be constructed in which a pixel is blacked out when that pixel's fundamental frequency curve is maximally positive. This frame number is computed from the phase matrix by:

$$F = R \ (1 + P(N - 1)/360).$$

F is the frame number, R is a rounding-off function used to make F an integer, N is the total number of frames desired for the cinematic display and P is the phase in degrees. Only those pixels of which the first harmonic amplitude is above a certain threshold are displayed in this manner. This display of the phases is superimposed either over the original EGNA study or over the amplitude image to serve as an anatomical guide and can be displayed as a cinematic endless loop. While providing a very attractive display, the whole procedure gives no more detailed information than an adequate representation of the phase matrix (Fig.18).

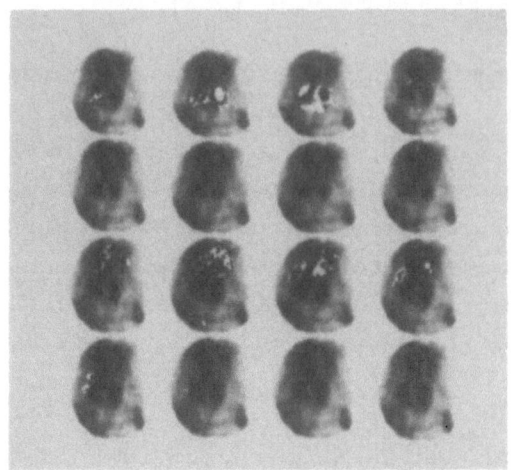

Fig. 18. Display of the wave of emptying.

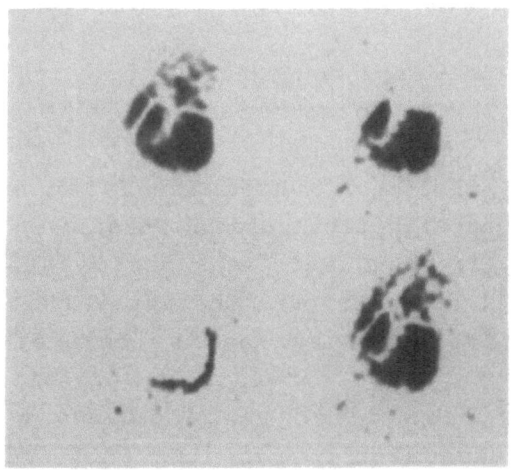

Fig. 19. Comparison of amplitude image with other functional
images.
u.l. : amplitude
u.r. : regional stroke volume
l.l. : regional ejection fraction
l.r. : composite stroke volume

## 4.5. COMPARISON WITH OTHER FUNCTIONAL IMAGES

The diagnostic use of functional imaging procedures is often limited due to the high noise content of the scintigraphic data which propagates into the functional images. Conventional functional imaging procedures of studies are related to parameters which describe the change in activity of each pixel between end diastole (ED) and end systole (ES). Figure 19 compares for the same EGNA study the amplitude image with a regional stroke volume (RSV) image, a regional ejection fraction (REF) image (15) and a composite stroke volume (CSV) image. The latter parameters were calculated as follows :

$$SV = ED - ES \qquad \text{if } ED - ES < 0 \qquad \text{the pixel is set 0}$$
$$EF = (ED - ES)/ED \qquad \text{if } ED - ES < 0 \qquad \text{the pixel is set 0}$$
$$CSV = |ED - ES|$$

The amplitude image compares best with a CSV image. The CSV image has been proposed as most accurately delineating left and right ventricular areas (16). Experimentally however, the amplitude image shows consistently less noise as compared to the other functional images.

## 4.6. CONTRIBUTION OF HIGHER HARMONICS

The spectrum resulting from a Fourier transform of an EGNA study in a normal person usually shows a dominant first harmonic, together with substantial contributions of higher harmonics (Fig.20). The information content of the series can be evaluated from the power density function which consists of the amplitude in the Fourier spectrum squared, hence most of the dynamic information is evidently found in the first harmonic.

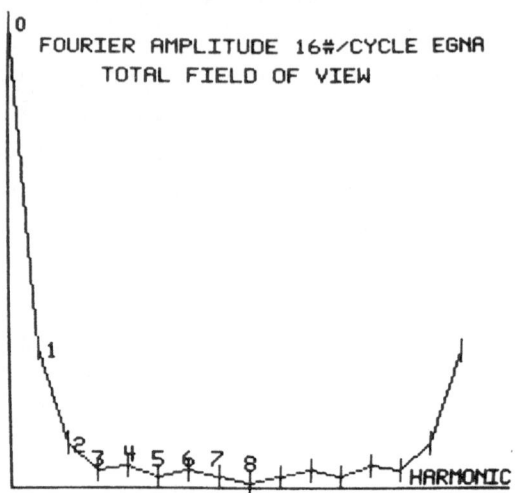

Fig. 20.  Fourier spectrum of EGNA study.

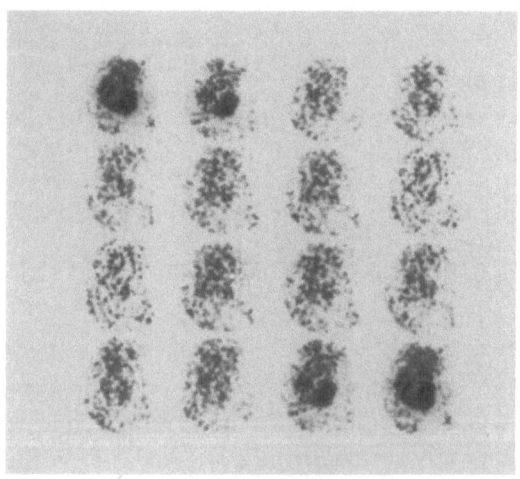

Fig. 21.  Higher harmonic amplitudes of 16 frame EGNA study.

In our approach, the basic frequency in the Fourier spectrum equals the average heart cycle frequency. The spatial distribution of the information discarded can be studied by displaying higher harmonic amplitudes and phases as functional images (Fig. 21). As the relative contribution of the higher harmonics is at least in part due to the asymmetry in the time/activity curves, we investigated the effects of cycle length on the second harmonic amplitude and phase images. The data from one subject with a long flat diastasis period (HR 60/min.) were analysed at the basic frequency equal to the heart frequency and after omitting 5 images from the end of the cardiac cycle (Fig.22). When the basic period equals the heart period, a substantial amount of information is still displayed in the second harmonic images. If the basic period is varied to exclude the diastasis frames, the power in the higher harmonics can be reduced (17). At the present time no experimental data are available which allow to attribute a specific physiological interpretation to the information present in the second or higher harmonics. The introduction of higher harmonics has well been used as an alternative narrow band pass filter in time (18,19,20).

## 4.7. SYSTEMATIC ERROR INTRODUCED BY GATING ARTEFACT

A subjects at rest in normal rhythm will exhibit fluctuations in heart rate which can cause a distortion in the late diastolic period of the averaged cardiac cycle. If some beats are slightly shorter than others, the last image of the sequence will contain fewer counts than the rest of the images. When the original data are not corrected for this distortion, stationary background is no longer eliminated from the amplitude/phase images. Similarly such gating artefacts also deteriorate the first harmonic

sinusoid approximation within the heart region. Therefore,
as part of the preprocessing, the original data series is
corrected for these distortions. Provided that the whole
heart region is within the field of view of the gamma
camera, that no other pulsating blood pool exists (e.g.
liver in tricuspid regurgitation (21) and that no gamma-ray
absorption is present, the total number of counts of each
individual frame should remain constant during the averaged
cardiac cycle. The correction for gating artefact can
therefore consists in equalisation of the total count rate
in each image (Fig.23). The most reliable way of correction
however takes into account the true measurement of time for
each frame. These time measurements should be determined
with 0.1 msec. resolution according to reference 20.

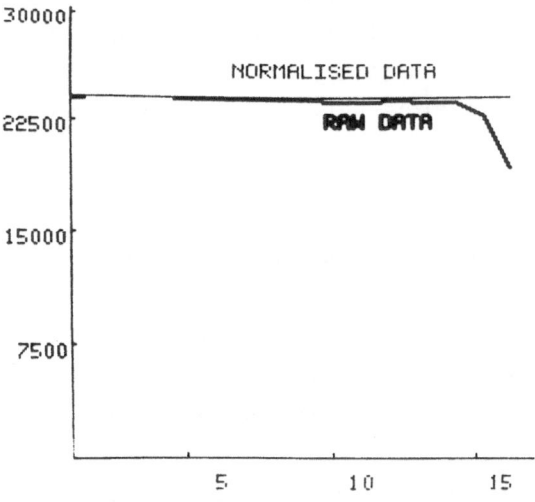

Fig. 23. Correction of gating artefacts - effect on
stationary structure.

4.8. DISCUSSION

Although the information content of EGNA studies as
compared to other scintigraphic techniques is very high,
image contrast, photon noise and sampling frequency limit
the visual extraction of relevant temporal information. The
detectability of patterns in timing and magnitude of count
rate variations in the images is a function of the
psychophysical properties of our vision. Due to this, when
EGNA images are displayed in cine mode, information on 4
dimensional regional cardiac performance (volume changes in
time) is mostly limited to the inspection of the ventricular
edges. Functional imaging procedures overcome some of these
limitations by data reduction and pattern extraction.

The evaluation of cardiac function from count rate
derived functional images has the advantage to rely upon a
more fundamental aspect of the tracer technique rather than
upon a pure morphological interpretation. A TFT takes into
account the information content of the whole cardiac cycle
for the calculation of the functional images. This is not
the case for other count rate derived functional images such
as the SV, REF or paradox image (22,15,23), in which data
processing is reduced to the information content in ED and
ES frames. As a result, the amplitude and phase images
provide a powerful means to improve the interpretation of
the EGNA studies in terms of time and space resolution.

Since each pixel's time activity curve is approximated
by a single frequency sine wave, the accuracy of the
amplitude/phase functional images will depend on the
contribution of the first harmonic to the information
content of the whole Fourier spectrum. It has been shown,
theoretically and experimentally, that the influence of
various diastolic as well as systolic components in the

54

shape of the left ventricular time/activity curve influence
the corresponding amplitude and phase complex (24, 25). The
implicit assumption of symmetry in the first harmonic model
prevents one from unequivocally determining which component
of the contraction/relaxation cycle is delayed. However, as
a functional mapping procedure of a pixel's time/activity
curve shape influenced by many or all of these components, a
TFT still proves useful in  separating abnormal subjects
from individuals with normal cardiac function.


REFERENCES

1.  Hoffmann  C.,  Kleine  W.  1965.  Eine neue Methode  zur
    unblutigen  Messung des Schlagvolumens am Menschen  uber
    viele  Tage mit Hilfe von  Radioaktive  Isotopen.  Verb.
    Dtsch. Ges. Kreislaufforsch. 31, 93.
2.  Zaret B.L.,  Strauss H.W.,  Hurley P.L.  et al. 1971. A
    noninvasive  scintiphotographic  method  for  detecting
    regional dysfunction in man.  New  Engl.  J.  Med.  284,
    1165.
3.  Parker J.A.,  Secker-Walker R.,  Hill R. et al. 1972. A
    new  technique  for the calculation of left  ventricular
    ejection fraction. J.Nucl.Med. 13, 649.
4.  Green M.V., Ostrow H.G., Douglas M.A. et al. 1975. High
    temporal  resolution  ECG-gated  scintigraphic
    angiocardiography. J.Nucl.Med. 16, 95.
5.  Bacharach S.L.,  Green M.V.,  Borer J.S. et al. 1977. A
    real-time  system for multi-image gated cardiac studies.
    J.Nucl.Med. 18, 79.
6.  Wagner H.N.,  Wake R.,  Nickoloff E.  et al.  1976. The
    Nuclear Stethoscope:  A simple device for generation of
    left ventricular volume curves. Am. J. Cardiol. 38, 747.
7.  Bacharach S.L., Green M.V., Borer S.J. et al. 1977. ECG-
    Gated  Scintillation  Probe  Measurement  of  Left
    Ventricular Function. J. Nucl. Med. 18, 1176.
8.  De Graaf C.N., Van Rijck P.P., Jambroes G. et al. 1977.
    Functional  imaging in nuclear cardiac studies.  IEEE  -
    Computers in Cardiology, 9.
9.  Adam  W.E.,  Tarkowska  A.,  Bitter  F.  et  al.  1977.
    Equilibrium  (gated)  radionuclide  ventriculography.
    Cardiovascular Radiology 2, 161.
10. Bossuyt A.,  Deconinck F., Lepoudre R. et al. 1979. The
    temporal  Fourier  transform  applied  to  functional
    isotopic imaging. In : Information Processing in Medical
    Imaging - INSERM 88, 397.

11. Pavel D., Zimmer A.M., Patterson V.N. 1977. In vivo labeling of red blood cells with 99m-Tc. A new approach to blood pool visualisation.J.Nucl.Med. 18, 305.
12. De Graaf C.N., Van Rijck P.P. 1976. High temporal and high phase resolution construction techniques for cardiac motion imaging. In : Medical Radionuclide Imaging - IAEA-SM, 337.
13. Verba J.W., Bornstein I., Alazraki N.P. et al. 1979. Onset and progression of mechanical systole derived from gated radionuclide techniques and displayed in cine format. J.Nucl.Med. 20, 625.
14. Links J.M., Douglas H.K., Wagner H.N. 1980. Patterns of ventricular emptying by Fourier analysis of gated blood pool studies J.Nucl.Med. 21, 978.
15. Maddox D.E., Holman B.L., Wyne J. et al. 1978. A noninvasive index of regional left ventricular wall motion. Am. J. Cardiol. 41, 1230.
16. Rigo P., Alderson P.O., Robertson R.M. et al. 1979. Measurement of aortic and mitral regurgitation by gated cardiac blood pool scans. Circulation 60, 306.
17. Vos P., Vossepoel A., Beekhuis H. et al. 1980. Characterisation of the ventricular function by temporal Fourier transform of gated blood pool studies. Nucl. Med. Comm. 1, 10.
18. King M.A., Doherty P.W. 1982. Cardiac image processing using an array processor. In: Digital Imaging Clinical Advances in Nuclear Medicine. Esser P.D. (Ed.) 153.
19. Goris M.L., Briandet P.A., Kriss J.P. 1982. Decomposition of the information content of first harmonic phase images. In: Nuclear Medicine and Biology Raynaud C.(Ed.) 46.
20. Bitter F., Adam W.E., Geffers H. et al. 1979. Synchronised steady state heart investigation. In : Proc. Inter. Symp. Fundamentals in Technical Progress. Vol.III, 9.1
21. Pavel D.G., Handler B., Lam W. et al. 1981. A new method for detection of tricuspidinsufficiency.J. Nucl. Med. 22, P4.
22. Itti R., Planiol T., Pellois A. 1975. Cardiac functional imaging from cinescintigraphic data. In : Information Processing in Scintigraphy. Raynaud C., Todd-Pokropek (Eds), 174.
23. Holmann B.L., Wyne J., Idoine J. et al. 1979. The paradox image : a noninvasive index of regional left ventricular dyskinesis. J.Nucl.Med. 20, 1237.
24. Bacharach S., De Graaf C., Van Rijck P. et al. 1981. Fourier phase distribution maps in the left ventricle of normal subjects at rest and exercise. In: Functional mapping of organ systems and other topics. Esser P. (Ed.) 139.
25. Wendt III R.E., Murphy P.H., Clark J.W. et al. 1982. Interpretation of Multigated Fourier Functional Images. J. Nucl. Med. 23, 715.

5. CLINICAL EVALUATION OF AMPLITUDE/PHASE ANALYSIS FOR THE ASSESSMENT OF REGIONAL WALL MOTION DISTURBANCES.

## 5.1. INTRODUCTION

Coronary arteriography and contrast ventriculography are the standard techniques by which coronary morphology and ventricular pump function are evaluated in patients with CAD. Both are invasive procedures which require catheterisation. They are associated with a significant degree of morbidity (1) and their radiation burden is not negligible (2). Serial cardiac catheterisations to determine the effect of medical and surgical treatment are therefore impractical. Radionuclide ventriculography (RNV) is non invasive and results in a radiation burden reduced by a factor 10 (3). The major clinical applications of RNV therefore are the repeated evaluation of ventricular performance in the follow-up of patients with heart disease, in monitoring physiologic or therapeutic intervention studies and in the evaluation of critically ill patients (4).

In order to assess objectively the effects of therapeutic interventions and disease on ventricular performance, the clinical evaluation of regional wall motion disturbances (RWMD) should fulfill the following requirements :

- low detectability threshold,
- localisation of the asynergic region in function of the affected coronary arteries,
- evaluation of the severity of the disturbance.

The term "asynergy" was first used by Harrison (5) to describe segments of the left ventricular wall demonstrating disorganised contraction. Herman (6,7,) subsequently introduced the terms hypokinetic, akinetic and dyskinetic to describe the degree of asynergy. Hypokinetic segments contract less vigorously than normal. Akinetic segments do not contract, while dyskinetic segments move outwardly or paradoxically during systole (Fig.24).

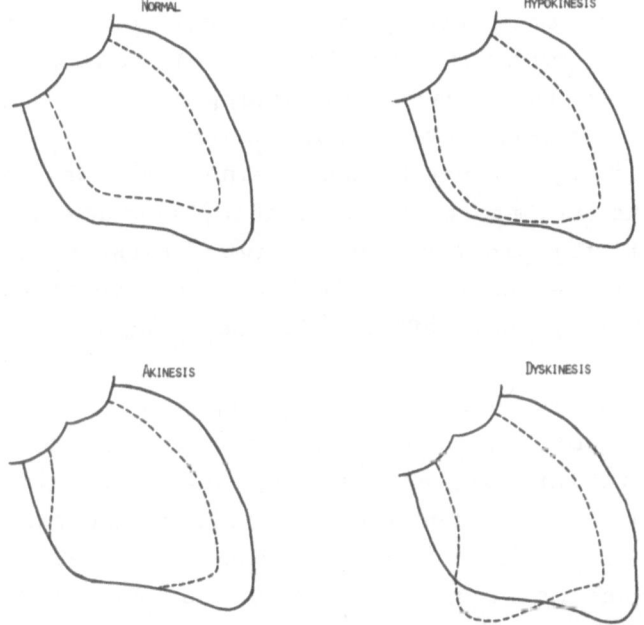

Fig.24. Schematic representation of end diastolic (solid line) and end systolic (dashed line) silhouettes of left ventricular cineangiograms.

## 5.2. EFFECT OF RWMD ON AMPLITUDE AND PHASE

Disturbances in regional myocardial contractility result in decreased and delayed blood volume changes in the corresponding part of the ventricle. Amplitude and phase images will allow the diagnosis and location of RWMD as defective regions in a left ventricle which is normally expected to contract homogeneously.

This is illustrated in an EGNA study of a patient with a huge antero-apical aneurysm, that showed a paradoxical motion on a recurrent movie display (Fig.25). Figure 25.a. represents the preprocessed original data series. Figure 25.b. represents the end diastolic and end systolic frames. Two ROI were determined : one corresponds to the normal contracting part of the left ventricle, the other corresponds to the paradoxical moving apex. Within each of these ROI, time/activity curves and their respective approximation by a first harmonic sine wave were determined. There exists an important phase delay between both curves. As a result, the blood volume changes in the antero-apical segment no longer contribute to the effective stroke volume. On the contrary, their effect will be opposite.

Figure 25.c. represents the amplitude and the phase images, the amplitude/phase distribution within a global left ventricular ROI, and the regional ejection fraction (REF) image. The distribution of amplitude and phases within the left ventricle is bimodal. The localisation and the extent of the asynergic region can be evaluated from the functional images. In the antero-apical region we distinguish an area with relatively decreased amplitude delineated from the rest of left ventricle by a margin wherein no or little changes occur. The phase image defines the region as dyskinetic as there exists a phase shift of

more than 90° with respect to the rest of the left
ventricle. The REF image does not allow the delineation of
the borders of the dyskinetic area. This is possible with
amplitude and phase images. Higher harmonic amplitude and
phase images give no additional clinical information (Fig.
25.d.).


## 5.3.  EFFECT  OF THE LOCALISATION OF RWMD ON  AMPLITUDE  AND PHASE

Without tomographic reconstruction, gamma-camera images
represent a two dimensional projection of a three
dimensional distribution of activity. As a result, even in a
normal homogeneously contracting ventricle, the amplitude
image is not homogeneous. Figure 26 shows a transverse
section through the left ventricle in a plane perpendicular
to the gamma camera. The hatched border corresponds to the
volume changes between end diastole and end systole. In a
normal contracting ventricle, the projection of the
amplitudes has 2 maxima, determined by the ventricular
border in systole. The minimum in the center is a function
of global ejection fraction and becomes relatively more
important in case of diminished global ventricular function.
Experimentally, in LAO position, there exists a ring of
maxima in the amplitude image which is determined by the
border of the left ventricle in systole (Fig.17.c in Ch.4).

In the presence of tangentially located RWMD, the
aspect of the amplitude images changes with the severity of
the asynergy. A dyskinetic area is characterised by a border
of zero amplitude and a new increase in amplitude at the
periphery. For non tangential hypo- or akinetic areas,
differentiation from global hypocontractility is no longer
possible on the basis of the amplitude image alone, whereas
dyskinetic areas still have a characteristic pattern.

60

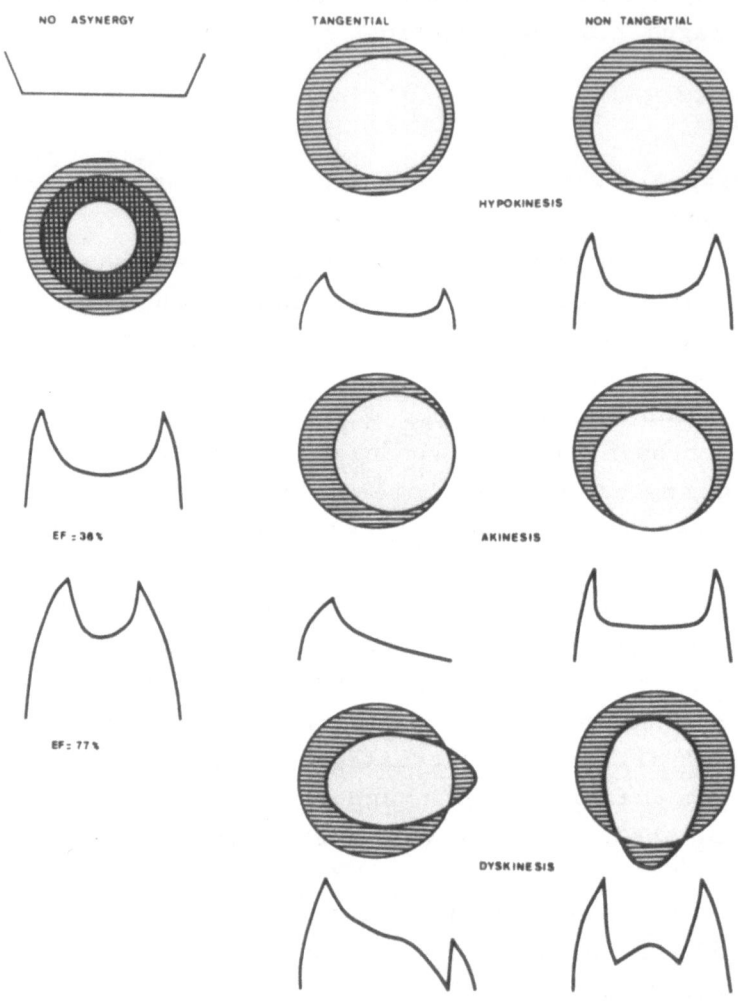

Fig. 26. Effect of the localisation of RWMD on the amplitude
         image.

The phase image is less influenced by the localisation of the asynergic region, although the importance of a phase shift also tends to be lessened by superposition of normal contracting regions. As

$$\cos (\omega t + \phi_1) + \cos (\omega t + \phi_2) = 2 \cos (\frac{\phi_1 - \phi_2}{2}) \cos (\omega t + \frac{\phi_1 + \phi_2}{2})$$

the superposition of 2 regions with a different phase does not introduce higher harmonics, in the first harmonic model.

5.4. CRITERIA FOR THE ASSESSMENT OF RWMD FROM AMPLITUDE/ PHASE IMAGES

As in theory one should expect that the volume changes occuring with a phase shift of more than 90. no longer contribute to the effective stroke volume, we describe areas with a phase delay of more than 90° as corresponding to dyskinetic motion. A phase delay below 90° is interpreted as hypo- or, by extrapolation, akinetic. The succession of colors in the cyclic color code is adapted such that in patients with normal rhythm a phase delay of 90° is represented in red contrasting with the green yellow of the normal part of the ventricles.

Examples of RWMD with increasing severity and different localisation in the left or right ventricle are shown in figure 29. As, at equilibrium, blood volume changes occuring during an averaged cardiac cycle are visualised for both ventricles, the assessment of right ventricular RWMD is possible as well.

## 5.5. COMPARISON WITH CONTRAST VENTRICULOGRAPHY

### 5.5.1. Methodology

To validate the clinical utility of the functional imaging procedure, RWMD determined from EGNA studies were compared to the information available from contrast ventriculography.

The study group consisted of 116 patients who all underwent cardiac catheterisation with coronary arteriography and contrast angiography as part of routine clinical evaluation of CAD. Contrast angiographies were evaluated by a single observer, independently of the results of the radionuclide studies. Single plane left ventricular cineangiography was carried out in 45. RAO and if possible 15 minutes later in 45. LAO positions, allowing "biplane" evaluation of regional wall motion. Regional wall motion was evaluated from superimposed outlines of the cavity silhouettes drawn at end diastole and end systole. Specific segments were determined according to the recommendations of the AHA (8). Fourteen subjects had near normal coronary arteriography (stenoses smaller than 50%) and normal contrast ventriculography. 102 had at least one stenosis larger than 50% of one of the three main coronary arteries : left anterior descending (LAD), circumflex (Cx) or right coronary artery (RCA). EGNA was performed as described in 4.2. A total of $6 \times 10^6$ counts were recorded over the whole averaged cardiac cycle. No change in the patients clinical status occured between the radionuclide study and the contrast ventriculography.

For each radionuclide study, polaroid exposures of
amplitude and phase images and the amplitude modulated phase
distribution histogram in the left ventricle were examined
for RWMD. Studies were classified according to the detection
and localisation of asynergy in 5 regions : anteroseptal
(AS), anterior-anterolateral (A-AL), apical (AP),
posterobasal (PB) and posterolateral (PL). The criteria used
to define the localisation of RWMD in a modified LAO view
are shown in figure 30.

Right ventricle                    Left ventricle

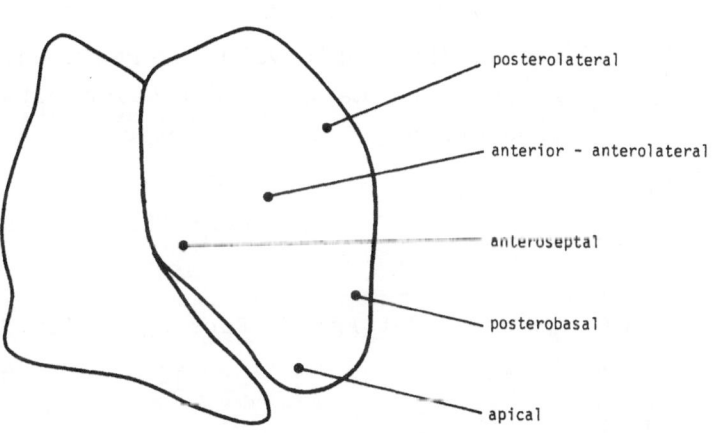

Fig.30. Localisation of RWMD in a modified LAO view.

## 5.5.2. Results

Table 1 shows the global diagnostic value of the functional imaging procedure for the detection and localisation of RWMD in the 116 patients with contrast angiography taken as standard. 69 patients were considered as abnormal and 40 as normal by both techniques. Two patients with normal contrast angiography had an abnormal RNV, one of them had ECG signs of diaphragmatic infarction. 5/74 patients with an abnormal contrast angiography had normal amplitude and phase images. A complete agreement with respect to the location of all segmental wall motion disturbances was found in 42/74 patients (57%). Whereas in 18/74 (24%) there was only a partial agreement. In 9/74 patients, both techniques disagreed completely with respect to the localisation of asynergy. When only the diagnosis normal/abnormal wall motion was considered, the sensitivity of radionuclide studies was 93% (64/74), the specificity 95% (40/42).

Table 1. Global diagnostic value of radionuclide ventriculography for the differentiation between normal and abnormal regional wall motion.

| RADIONUCLEDY | ANGIOGRAPHY | | CONTRAST ANGIOGRAPHY | | | |
|---|---|---|---|---|---|---|
| | | | | AN | | N |
| | | | Tot.Agr. | Part.Agr. | Tot.Disagr. | |
| | AN | AN | 42 | 18 | 9 | 2 |
| | N | N | | | 5 | 40 |

Complete Agreement : 42/74 (57 %)
Partial  Agreement : 18/74 (25 %)

Table 2 gives in detail the comparison between the dysynergic areas observed by both techniques. Taking into consideration that both septal (S) and anterior-anterolateral (A-AL) areas are perfused by branches of the same coronary artery (CAD), we found agreement between both techniques in 84/111 regions (75%). Most of the discrepancies were observed for contractility disturbances located in non tangential segments on radionuclide angiography. At the opposite, septal wall motion anomalies were better evidenced on radionuclide angiography. However, this may be explained by the fact that in 32 patients, coronary arteriography was performed in RAO and LL positions instead of RAO and LAO positions, the first one being less sensitive to septal anomalies. A very good agreement was observed so far as global hypocontractility is concerned.

Table 2. Comparison between radionuclide ventriculography and contrast ventriculography for the assessment of regional wall motion disturbances with respect to their localisation.

CONTRAST ANGIOGRAPHY

RADIONUCLIDE ANGIOGRAPHY

| | S (LAD) | A-AL (LAD) | AP (LAD,RCA) | PB/PL (RCA,Cx) | GH | N |
|---|---|---|---|---|---|---|
| S(LAD) | 10 | 4 | 4 | | | 2 |
| AL(LAD) | 2 | 16 | 1 | | | 1 |
| AP(LAD,RCA) | | 1 | 33 | 2 | | 2 |
| PL(RCA,Cx) | | 4 | 2 | 19 | | |
| GH | | | | | 7 | |
| N | | 4 | 3 | 5 | | |

When the severity of RWMD was evaluated according to Hamilton (9), most discrepancies were observed in the classes of patients with either localised hypo- or akinesis or localised dyskinesis (Table 3). It should be stressed that the evaluation of both techniques was subjective. Nevertheless, these discrepancies are mainly due to the fact that we used the criterion of phase shift greater or smaller than 90° to differentiate between dyskinesis and hypo- or akinesis.

Table 3. Comparison between radionuclide ventriculography and contrast ventriculography for the evaluation of the severity of RWMD.

CONTRAST VENTRICULOGRAPHY

| RADIONUCLIDE ANGIOGRAPHY | 0 | 1 | 2 | 3 | 4 |
|---|---|---|---|---|---|
| 0 | 40 | 1 | 4 | | |
| 1 | 1 | 2 | | | |
| 2 | | | 27 | 8 | |
| 3 | | | 9 | 16 | |
| 4 | | | | | 7 |

Class 0: normal left ventricular function
1: borderline abnormal
2: localised hypo- or akinesis
3: localised dyskinesis
4: diffuse a- or hypokinesis

## 5.6. DISCUSSION

It is demonstrated in this chapter that regional contractility can readily be determined by functional imaging of cardiac blood pool studies. RWMD is studied here in terms of regional count rate changes, which are supposed to be linearly related to the regional blood volume changes. They are described in an orthogonal coordinate system with reference points external to the heart. As such, the isotopic approach is conceptually different from the geometric descriptions of ventricular contours in radiographic studies (10,11,12,13,14). Several limiting factors have to be taken into account while interpreting RWMD from amplitude/phase images. The "normal" amplitude image is not homogeneous, especially in the right heart side, where the displacement of RA and RV during the cardiac cycle are responsible for the low amplitude area corresponding to the superimposition of the RA and RV on the projected image. In general, overlap of intra- and extraventricular structures affect the maps. These problems however are inherent to the acquisition procedure and in fact are only much more clearly apparent in amplitude/phase displays than with other data processing procedures.

In routine clinical use, comparison of the results obtained by radionuclide and radiographic studies reveals two discrepancies :

1. With respect of the exact localisation of RWMD, non tangential segments are less well visualised on radionuclide ventriculography, in particular when they are hypokinetic. Although wall motion disturbances in non tangential segments could be detected from a single LAO view, the accuracy of their localisation increased when data were acquired from two views (14). This becomes more important when more than

one asynergic segment was present. A more accurate assessment of the exact localisation of RWMD would require tomographic reconstruction. In addition to the evaluation of left ventricular contractility, EGNA studies allow the objectivation of right ventricular disturbances. Radiographic evaluation of right ventricular dysfunction would necessitate a supplementary right catheterisation.

2. With respect of the severity of RWMD, no good correlation was found between a paradoxical extension of the ventricular borders on contrast ventriculography and a more than 90° first harmonic phase delay of the blood volume changes. In the cineangiographic studies, the severity of regional abnormalities were described in terms of amplitude of motion of the left ventricular silhouette between end diastole and end systole. Abnormalities in the sequence of wall motion are less well appreciated on cineangiographic films (15). A severe methodological limitation to the present study is the subjective interpretation of both the contrast ventriculography and the functional images. A standardised evaluation of the severity of RWMD would require quantitative parameters.

The use of amplitude/phase imaging in clinical practice introduces the concept that regional contractility can be described in terms of two independent variables : magnitude and timing of contraction. In the TFT applied here, the temporal model is restricted to the first harmonic changes in activity. In this situation, amplitude and phase characterise the whole cyclic phenomenon. Their combined use improves the diagnostic performance of RNV for the assessment of RWMD.

REFERENCES

1.  Adams F. 1973. The complications of coronary arteriography. Circulation 48, 609.
2.  Ardran G.M., Hamill J., Emrys-Roberts E. et al. 1970. Radiation dose to the patient in cardiac radiology. Brit. J.Radiol. 43, 391.
3.  Smith A. 1965. Internal dose calculation for 99m-Tc. J.Nucl.Med. 6, 231.
4.  Berger H.J., Zaret B.L. 1981. Nuclear Cardiology (second of two parts). New Engl. J. Med. 15, 855.
5.  Harrison T.R. 1965. Some unanswered questions concerning enlargement and failure of heart. Am. Heart J. 69, 100.
6.  Herman M.V., Heile R.A., Klein M.D. et al. 1967. Localised disorders of myocardial contraction. New Engl. J. Med. 227, 222.
7.  Herman M.V., Gorlin R. 1969. Implications of left ventricular asynergy. Am. J. Cardiol. 23, 538.
8.  Austen G., Edwards J., Frye R. et al. 1975. A reporting system on patients evaluated for coronary artery disease. Circulation 51, 5A.
9.  Hamilton G.W., Murray J.A., Kennedy J.W. 1972. Quantitative angiocardiography in ischemic heart disease. The spectrum of abnormal left ventricle and the role of abnormally contracting segments. Circulation 45. 1065.
10. Adam W.E., Tarkowska F., Bitter F. et al. 1979. Equilibrium (gated) radionuclide ventriculography. Cardiovascular Radiology 2, 161.
11. Block P., Bossuyt A., Deconinck F. et al. 1979. Evaluation of a new technique of radionuclide angiography for the assessment of regional wall motion abnormalities. IEEE - Computers in Cardiology, 21.
12. Bossuyt A., Deconinck F., Block P. et al. 1979. Improved assessment of regional wall motion disturbances by temporal Fourier transform. Invest. Radiol. 14, 391.
13. Bossuyt A., Deconinck F., Demoor D. et al. 1981. Application of a temporal Fourier transform for evaluation of regional wall motion disturbances by radionuclide ventriculography at rest and during exercise. Acta Cardiologica Suppl. 26, 105.
14. Bossuyt A., Deconinck F., Prihadi J. et al. 1982. Contribution of radionuclide ventriculography for the assessment of regional wall motion anomalies at rest. Comparison with contrast ventriculography. In: Non Invasive Methods in Ischemic Heart Disease G. Faivre (Ed.) 35
15. Leighton R.F., Nelson A.D., Andrews L.T. 1979. Altered sequence of regional left ventricular wall motion in patients with coronary heart disease. IEEE - Computers in Cardiology, 149.

6. NON-INVASIVE ASSESSMENT OF THE PROXIMAL STENOSES OF THE
   MAIN CORONARY ARTERIES BY MEANS OF EXERCISE RADIONUCLIDE
   VENTRICULOGRAPHY


6.1. INTRODUCTION

In 1935, Tennant and Wiggers demonstrated that the
segment of myocardium supplied by an experimentally occluded
coronary artery would expand during systole. Experimentally,
regional mechanical performance has been shown to decrease
with the reduction of regional coronary flow. Clinically it
has been shown that asynergy, defined as regional wall
motion disturbances (RWMD), is usually related to
significant coronary artery disease (1, 2). When present at
rest, asynergy usually results from myocardial infarction
although it may also be present without evidence of
necrosis. In the latter case, the asynergic area can be
reversible and could be related to transient myocardial
ischemia (3,4). In CAD patients, contrast angiography and
radionuclide ventriculography (RNV) under stress may reveal
asynergic areas not always present at rest (5,6).

In the original exercise RNV studies the response of
the left ventricular ejection fraction to exercise was used
as a predictor of the presence of significant CAD
(7,8,9,10). RWMD induced in the same circumstances provided
either adjunctive or confirmative information. This study
investigates to what extent resting and exercise RNV could
contribute to the identification of the proximal stenoses of
the main coronary arteries by evidencing asynergy. The

results of stress RNV are compared with those obtained by exercise ECG and $^{201}$Tl myocardial perfusion scintigraphy (11, 12).

## 6.2. METHODS

### 6.2.1. Patient population and study protocol

Exercise RNV was performed in 8 normal subjects and in 52 male patients (36-66 y), submitted to coronary angiography with left ventriculography because of chest pain, compatible but not necessarily typical for angina pectoris. 24 of the patients had clinical evidence of previous myocardial infarction (MI). Table 1 gives in detail the coronary lesions objectivated in the patient population.

Table 1. Coronary lesions observed in the patient population

```
22 significative st. on LAD+Cx+RCA (or MTLCA+RCA)(15ˣ)(12MI)
 7       "       "   "   LAD + Cx (or MTLCA)        (6ˣ)(2 MI)
 4       "       "   "   LAD                        (4ˣ)(1 MI)
 2       "       "   "   Cx (1 with st. RCA . 50%)  (2ˣ)(1 MI)
 6       "       "   "   RCA (1 with 1 st. on S₁)   (3ˣ)(1 MI)
 6       "       "   "   RCA + Cx                   (3ˣ)(2 MI)
 5       "       "   "   RCA + LAD                  (4ˣ)(4 MI)
```

Legend : $S_1$  :  first septal branch of the LAD ;
         $^x$   :  number of patients with Tl scintigraphy ;
       x MI:  number of patients with evidence of previous myocardial infarction

The 12 conventional ECG leads and $^{201}$Tl myocardial scintigraphy images were recorded during a maximal or symptom limited standardised exercise test on bicycle ergometer as described by Lenaers (13). Subsequently, equilibrium gated cardiac blood pool studies were performed during the steady state of a submaximal exercise test carried out in supine position in order to reach a heart frequency of about 85% of the maximal heart frequency attained during the first stress test.

## 6.2.3. Stress electrocardiography

The 12 conventional ECG leads including $D_1$, $D_2$, $D_3$, aVR, aVL, aVF, $V_{1-6}$ were recorded every minute of the stress test and during the first 5 minutes of recovery. The localisation of the abnormal myocardial segments was postulated from the leads evidencing anomalies using the criteria of Table 2 (14).

Table 2.  ECG criteria for the localisation  of  myocardial segments.

| SEGMENTAL LOCALISATION | LEADS EVIDENCING ANOMALIES | | |
|---|---|---|---|
| Inferior septal (IS) | $D_{III}$ | aVF | $V_1$ |
| Anterior septal (AS) | $V_1$ | $V_2$ | |
| Apical          (AP) | $V_3$ | $V_4$ | |
| Lateral          (L) | $V_5$ | $V_6$ | |
| Posterior lateral | | | |
| High lateral (PL/HL) | $D_I$ | aVL | |
| Inferior         (I) | $D_{II}$ | $D_{III}$ | aVF |
| Posterior        (P) | $R\overline{V_1}$ | | |

## 6.2.3. Selective coronary angiography

Selective    coronary    arteriography    was    performed according  to  the technique  of  Judkins (15).  Arteriograms were   obtained   in at least left and right anterior  oblique (LAO,  RAO),  left lateral (LL) and cranio caudal positions. Only stenoses with a reduction of the diameter of the  lumen greater than 50% were considered significant.  The following arteries  were  examined : main trunk of the left  coronary artery  (MTLCA),  left  anterior  descending  artery  (LAD), artery  diagonalis (DIAG),  artery  circumflex  (Cx),  right coronary  artery (RCA).  Neither the length of the stenosis, nor the collateral circulation, nor the status of the distal bed  were taken into consideration as this proved to be  too complex.

## 6.2.4. Myocardial scintigraphy

Myocardial scintigraphy was performed by intravenous injection of 2 mCi $^{201}$Tl one minute before the end of the exercise test. Data acquisition was started within 10 minutes after the end of the exercise test and completed within the next 30 minutes. Images were obtained in LL, LAO (65, 45 and 25 degrees) and ANT positions. 200.000 counts were stored in each view. Spatial contrast enhancement is obtained by a 50% cut-off of the maximal LV activity determined after nine points smoothing. The 75% isocount level is outlined for easier evaluation of regional myocardial perfusion. Each segment is considered hypoperfused when the activity is below the 75% isocount level (13). The localisation of the segments on the myocardial perfusion images according to the nature of their irrigation is given in figure 31.

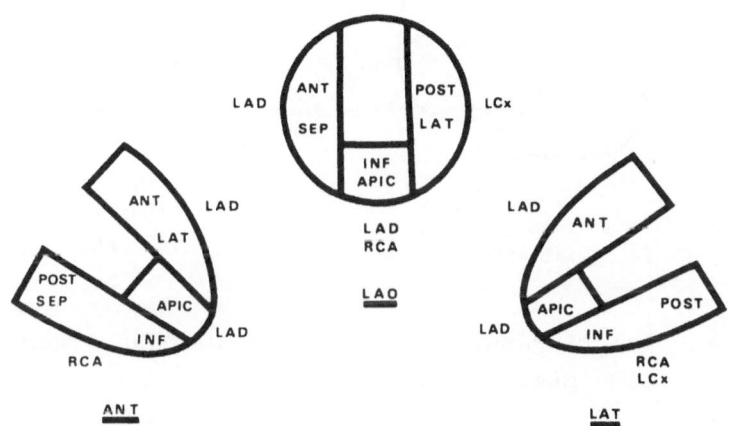

Fig. 31.   Scintigraphic localisation of myocardial perfusion defects and corresponding coronary arteries.

## 6.2.5. Radionuclide ventriculography

EGNA was performed in both anterior and LAO positions at rest and during submaximal exercise testing as described in Chapter 4.2. At each time data were accumulated during 3 minutes resulting in averaged cardiac cycles consisting of 150000 counts. For each study color polaroid exposures of amplitude and phase images and amplitude/phase distribution histograms within right and left ventricle (RV and LV) were examined for the presence of asynergy. Studies were classified according to the detection and the localisation of asynergy in the following regions : AS, IS, A-AL, AP, LA and PL. The criteria used in order to define the localisation of RWMD are shown in figure 32.

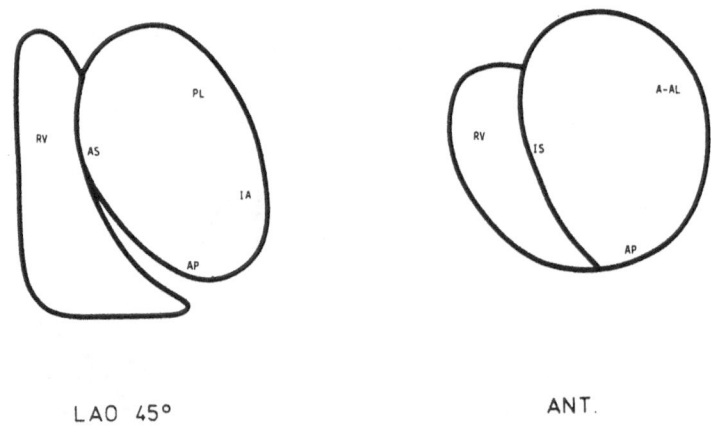

LAO 45°                              ANT.

Fig. 32. Scintigraphic localisation of RWMD in anterior and LAO images

## 6.2.6. Statistical analysis

Statistical analysis of the results was effectuated by the use of the Mc Nemar test. The criterion for significance was a probability (p) value of less than .05.

## 6.3. RESULTS

### 6.3.1. Comparative results of stress ECG and RNV

The results are summarized in Table 3. Only the ECG
anomalies recorded during the first maximal or symptom
limited stress test were taken into consideration. The
anomalies recorded during the second submaximal stress test
which served only for the recording of the exercise RNV
images, were not taken into account. The 8 normal subjects
all had a normal exercise RNV in spite of the presence of
ECG anomalies in 3 among them. In the group of patients with
CAD, exercise RNV gave significantly better results for the
assessment of significant stenoses of the lAD or the Cx
arteries by objectivating AS and PL RWMD at exercise.
However, there was no difference with respect to the
diagnosis of the RCA stenosis.

### 6.3.2. Comparative results of stress myocardial scintigraphy and RNV

As shown in Table 4, 2 among the normal subjects had
$^{201}$Tl fixation anomalies on the myocardial scintigraphy,
while the ventriculography was normal. In the group of 52
patients with CAD, exercise RNV gave significantly better
results for the assessment of significantly stenosed LAD
arteries, but there was no difference regarding the
identification of RCA or Cx stenoses. Nevertheless, the
specificity for RNV was higher than for myocardial
scintigraphy. Of the 119 wall segments with motion anomalies
on exercise RNV, 106 (89%) were hypoperfused on myocardial
scintigraphy, while 93 out of the 136 hypoperfused segments
had also motion anomalies. In any case, we found a closer
relationship between the anomalies evidenced by both
radionuclide techniques than with the type of the stenosed
arteries on the coronary arteriography.

| R + XECG | | | | | | | | CORONARY ARTERIOGRAPHY | RV at R + X | | | | | | | | |
|---|---|---|---|---|---|---|---|---|---|---|---|---|---|---|---|---|---|
| P | I | PL/HL | L | AP | AS | IS | N | | N | GH | IS | AS | AP | AL | PL | IA | RV |
| | | 3 | 2 | 1 | | | | NORMAL ($8^x$) | 8 | | | | | | | | |
| 3 | 12 | 11 | 13 | 10 | 10 | 5 | 2 | LAD + Cx + RCA ($22^x$) | 1 | 3 | 13 | 14 | 18 | 14 | 15 | 8 | 7 |
| | 2 | 3 | 2 | 2 | 5 | | 1 | LAD + Cx or MTLCA ($7^x$) | 1 | 1 | 2 | 4 | 6 | 4 | 3 | 2 | |
| | 2 | 2 | 3 | 3 | 1 | | | LAD ($4^x$) | | 1 | 1 | 2 | 3 | 3 | | 1 | |
| 2 | 1 | | 2 | 1 | 1 | | | Cx ($2^x$, with 1 st. RCA < 50%) | | | 2 | | 2 | | 2 | 1 | |
| 2 | 4 | 2 | 3 | 2 | | | 2 | RCA ($6^x$, 1 with 1 st. $S_1$) | 2 | | 2 | | 3 | | 4 | 2 | 5 |
| 2 | 1 | 2 | 1 | | 1 | 1 | 1 | RCA + Cx ($6^x$) | | | 1 | | 4 | 1 | 4 | 1 | 2 |
| 1 | 3 | 4 | 4 | | 4 | 2 | 1 | RCA + LAD ($5^x$) | 1 | | 4 | 4 | 5 | 3 | 4 | 3 | 3 |

Table 3. Comparison between ECG and RNV for the assessment of the number and type of stenosed arteries.

| Ex. MYOCARDIAL SCINTIGRAPHY | | | | | | | CORONARY ARTERIOGRAPHY | REST + Ex. RADIONUCLIDE VENTRIC. | | | | | | | | |
|---|---|---|---|---|---|---|---|---|---|---|---|---|---|---|---|---|
| PB | PL | A/AL | AP | AS | I-PS | N | | N | GH | IS | AS | AP | A-AL | PL | IA | RV |
|  |  |  | 2 | 1 | 1 | 6 | NORMAL ($8^X$) | 8 |  |  |  |  |  |  |  |  |
| 8 | 8 | 11 | 11 | 8 | 9 |  | LAD + Cx + RCA ($15^X$) |  | 1 | 8 | 8 | 13 | 11 | 12 | 6 | 5 |
| 2 | 2 | 6 | 5 | 3 | 1 |  | LAD + Cx or MTLCA ($6^X$) | 1 | 1 | 2 | 3 | 5 | 3 | 2 | 2 |  |
|  | 2 | 4 | 3 | 2 | 2 |  | LAD ($4^X$) |  |  | 1 | 2 | 3 | 3 |  | 1 |  |
|  | 2 | 1 | 2 |  | 1 |  | Cx ($2^X$, 1 with st. RCA < 50%) |  |  |  | 2 | 2 |  | 2 | 1 |  |
| 3 | 2 |  | 3 |  | 1 |  | RCA ($3^X$, 1 with st. $S_1$) |  |  | 1 |  | 2 |  | 3 | 1 | 3 |
| 3 | 3 | 2 | 3 |  | 1 |  | RCA + Cx ($3^X$) |  |  | 1 |  | 2 | 1 | 3 |  | 2 |
| 1 | 2 | 3 | 3 | 2 | 3 |  | RCA + LAD ($4^X$) |  |  | 3 | 3 | 4 | 2 | 1 | 2 | 1 |

Table 4. Comparison between stress myocardial perfusion scintigraphy and RNV for the assessment of the number and type of stenosed arteries

### 6.3.3. Global results

In this study, an abnormal rest or exercise RNV represented a higher specific (100%) and very sensitive (90%) finding for the diagnosis of coronary artery disease, even if the type of coronary involvement was not always correctly assigned.

The respective contribution of the 3 non-invasive techniques used for the assessment of the main stenosed coronary arteries are summarised in Table 5, 6 and 7. In our patient population we observed that :
- RNV was a very specific technique for the assessment of the type of main stenosed arteries, since there were only 10 false positives (global specificity : 86%).
- For the assessment of LAD stenosis, very good results were obtained by all 3 techniques, with however significantly better results for RNV.
- For the assessment of circumflex stenoses, poor results were observed with stress ECG, whereas both myocardial scintigraphy and RNV yielded significantly better results.
- No differences in sensitivity were observed with respect to the assessment of RCA stenosis.

The demonstration by RNV of right ventricular RWMD was highly specific for RCA stenosis (specificity : 100%), even if it was not sensitive (43%).

The predictive value of both positive and negative radionuclide images was high for the evaluation of the presence or absence of LAD or Cx stenosis. By contrast, it was much lower for the diagnosis of RCA stenosis. In this case, a negative image did not allow to exclude a significant stenosis of this artery, while a positive image was not typical for RCA stenosis (except when right ventricular RWMD were observed). Stress RNV allowed even in some cases to demonstrate isolated stenoses on the diagonal or septal branches of the left anterior descending artery.

Table 5. Diagnostic value of rest and exercise ECG for the assessment of the type of stenosed arteries.

| Number of stenosed arteries | | Rest and Exercise ECG + | - | $P_V+$ | $P_V-$ |
|---|---|---|---|---|---|
| LAD (38) | 38+ | 30 (75%) | 8 | 88 | 71 |
| | 24- | 4 | 20 (85%) | | |
| Cx (37) | 37+ | 16 (43%) | 21 | 66 | 45 |
| | 25- | 8 | 17 (68%) | | |
| RCA (39) | 39+ | 27 (69%) | 12 | 93 | 64 |
| | 23- | 2 | 21 (91%) | | |
| Total (194) | 114+ | 73 (64%) | 41 | | |
| | 72- | 14 | 58 (81%) | | |

Table 6. Diagnostic value of exercise myocardial scintigraphy

| Number of ste-nosed arteries | | Rest and Exercise ECG + | − | $P_V+$ | $P_V-$ |
|---|---|---|---|---|---|
| LAD (38) | 29+ | 24 (83%)[ns] | 5 | 92 | 66 |
| | 12− | 2 | 10 (83%)[ns] | | |
| Cx (37) | 25+ | 15 (60%)[x] | 10 | 79 | 54 |
| | 16− | 4 | 12 (75%)[ns] | | |
| RCA (39) | 26+ | 18 (69%)[ns] | 8 | 90 | 62 |
| | 15− | 2 | 13 (87%)[ns] | | |
| Total (194) | 80+ | 57 (71%)[ns] | 23 | | |
| | 43− | 8 | 35 (81%)[ns] | | |

Table 7. Diagnostic value of regional wall motion disturbances at rest and at exercise.

| Number of stenosed arteries | | Rest and Exercise ECG + | − | $P_V+$ | $P_V-$ |
|---|---|---|---|---|---|
| LAD (38) | 38+ | 34 (89%) | 4 | 94 | 85 |
| | 24− | 2 | 22 (92%) | | |
| Cx (37) | 37+ | 22 (60%) | 15 | 91 | 60 |
| | 25− | 2 | 23 (92%) | | |
| RCA (39) | 39+ | 27 (69%) | 12 | 82 | 59 |
| | 23− | 6 | 17 (74%) | | |
| Total (194) | 114+ | 83 (80%) | 31 | | |
| | 72− | 10 | 62 (86%) | | |

## 6.4. DISCUSSION

With the exception of the diagnosis of stenosis of the left anterior descending artery, the conventional 12 leads exercise ECG did not contribute to the assessment of proximal stenosis of the main coronary arteries. Myocardial scintigraphy at exercise had a diagnostic superiority over stress ECG for the identification of both CAD and Cx stenoses, but not for the assessment of RCA stenosis. The diagnostic superiority of stress myocardial scintigraphy in comparison with exercise ECG was less obvious than in a previous study (13). This may result from the fact that in this study 12 leads were recorded instead of 4 in the previous one, and also that 24 out of the 52 patients had a previous myocardial infarction with ECG sequelae.

The best results were observed with exercise radionuclide ventriculography, even if one considers that this last technique was performed during a submaximal exercise test. Significant differences were observed in the correct assessment of the stenosed LAD and Cx arteries, both with respect to sensitivity as well as to specificity. No significant differences were observed for the diagnosis of RCA stenosis. However, RNV is one of the rare techniques which can demonstrate wall motion anomalies of the right ventricle (15,16). As shown in this study, this method is very specific, even though it is not sensitive for RCA stenosis.

The present data do not allow to conclude that there exists a non-invasive technique which enables to assess correctly the type of stenosed arteries, particularly when more than one artery is involved. Indeed, although alterations in myocardial perfusion and regional contractility are both more prevalent in wall segments perfused by severely stenosed arteries, they are not always present. On the contrary, we also sometimes observed such anomalies in myocardial areas irrigated by vessels which were not severely stenosed. A better correlation was found between regional wall motion and myocardial perfusion anomalies than with the nature of the stenosed coronary arteries as it was demonstrated on coronary arteriography. Similar observations have already been reported for the surface ECG mapping technique (17). This may perhaps be explained by the fact that this study does not take into account the stenoses of the smaller arteries, the length of the stenoses, the degree of development of the collateral circulation nor the state of the distal bed (18,19). The degree of confidence in the interpretation of coronary arteriograms can also explain some discrepancies (20). Moreover, it is known that some thrombosed arteries may later be recanalised, which explains the normal coronary arteriography sometimes observed in patients with ECG sequelae of myocardial infarction (21). This may explain why 6% of the patients with demonstrated CAD had wall motion anomalies on both contrast radionuclide ventriculographies which did not correspond to related stenosed arteries.

Absence of RWMD at rest and at exercise means almost certainly absence of severe proximal stenoses on a main coronary artery. In any case they mean a well preserved myocardial function, especially when global left ventricular ejection fraction remains normal during exercise. Both rest/exercise myocardial perfusion scintigraphy and RNV could be used in association with stress ECG in order to ascertain whether borderline stenoses on the coronary arteriography are hemodynamically significant.

REFERENCES

1.  Herman  M.V.,  Gorlin  R.  1969.  Implications  of  left
    ventricular asynergy. Am.J.Cardiol.23, 538.
2.  Baxlay  W.A.,  Reevs  T.J.  1971.  Abnormal  regional
    myocardial  performance  in  coronary  artery  disease.
    Progr. Cardiovasc. Dis. 13, 405.
3.  Massie  B.,  Bottvinck E.,  Brundage B.  et  al.  1978.
    Relationship  of  regional  myocardial  perfusion  to
    segmental  wall  motion.  A  physiologic  basis  for
    understanding  the  presence  and  reversibility  of
    asynergy. Circulation 58, 1154.
4.  Bodenheimer M.M.,  Banka V.S., Herman G.E. et al. 1976.
    Reversibility  asynergy  :  histopathologic  and
    electrocardiographic  correlation  in  patients  with
    coronary artery disease. Circulation 53, 792.
5.  Sharma B., Goodwin J.F., Raphael M.J. et al. 1975. Left
    ventricular angiography on exercise : a new method of
    assessing  left ventricular function in ischaemic  heart
    disease. Brit. Heart J., 38, 59.
6.  Banka V.S.,  Bodenheimer M.M. et al. 1976. Intervention
    ventriculography :  comparative value of  nitroglycerin,
    post-extrasystolic  potentiation  or nitroglycerin  plus
    post-extrasystolic potentiation. Circulation 53, 632.
7.  Borer J.S.,  Bacharach S.L.,  Green M.V.  et al.  1977.
    Real-time  radionuclide  cineangiography  in  the  non-
    invasive  evaluation  of  global  and  regional  left
    ventricular  function  at  rest and during  exercise  in
    patients with coronary artery disease. New Engl. J. Med.
    296, 839.
8.  Bodenheimer M.M., Banka V.S., Fosshee C.M. et al. 1978.
    Detection  of coronary heart disease using  radionuclide
    determined ejection fraction at rest and during handgrip
    exercise.  Correlation  with  coronary  anatomy.
    Circulation 58, 640.
9.  Jengo J.A.,  Oren V.,  Conant R. et al. 1979. Effect of
    maximal exercise stress on left ventricular function  in
    patients  with coronary artery disease using first  pass
    radionuclide angiography. A rapid, noninvasive technique
    for  determining  ejection fraction and  segmental  wall
    motion. Circulation 59, 60.
10. Rerych  S.K.,  Schaz P.M.,  Newman G.E.  et  al.  1978.
    Cardiac  function at rest and during exercise in normals
    and in  patients with coronary heart disease. Evaluation
    by radionuclide angiocardiography. Ann. Surg. 187, 449.
11. Block P.  Bossuyt A, Dewilde Ph.  et  al.  1981.  Non-
    invasive  assessment of the proximal stenoses of the main
    coronary  arteries.  Comparative results of stress  ECG,
    myocardial  scintigraphy  and  exercise  radionuclide
    ventriculography.  IEEE  - Computers in  Cardiology,  63.

12. Bossuyt A., Deconinck F., Demoor D. et al. 1981. Application of a temporal Fourier transform for evaluation of regional wall motion disturbances by radionuclide ventriculography at rest and during exercise. Acta Cardiologica Suppl. 26, 105.
13. Lenaers A., Block P., Van Thiel E. et al. 1977. Segmental analysis of Tl-201 stress myocardial scintigraphy. J.Nucl.Med. 18, 509.
14. Simoons M.L., Block P. 1981. Towards the optimal lead system and optimal criteria for exercise electrocardiography. Am. J. Cardiol. 47, 1366.
15. Rigo P., Murray M., Taylor D.R. et al. 1975. Right ventricular dysfunction detected by gated scintigraphy in patients with acute inferior myocardial infarction. Circulation 52, 268.
16. Huyghens L., Depoorter I., Bossuyt A. et al. 1981. Aanwinsten in de diagnose van het akute myokardinfarkt van het rechter ventrikel. Nucleair Geneeskundig Bulletin 4, 151.
17. Block P., Lenaers A., Dewilde Ph. et al. 1977. Diagnostic value of surface mapping recordings registered at rest and during exercise. In : IEEE - Computers in Cardiology. Kipley K.L., Ostrow H.G. (Eds), 89.
18. Haaz W., Iskandrian A.S., Segal B.L. et al. 1980. Effects of coronary artery narrowing, collaterals and left ventricular function on the pattern of myocardial perfusion. Cathet. Cardiovasc. Diag. 6, 159.
19. Tubau J., Chaitman B., Bourassa M. et al. 1981. Importances of coronary collateral circulation in interpreting exercise test results. Am. J. Cardiol. 47, 27.
20. Zir L.M., Miller S.W., Dinsmore R.E. et al. 1976. Interobserver variability in coronary angiography. Circulation. 53, 627.
21. Bertiu A., Pare J.C., Sanz G.A. 1981. Myocardial infarction with normal coronary arteries: a prospective clinical angiographic study. Am. J. Cardiol. 48, 28.

7. FUNCTIONAL DISSIMILARITY BETWEEN ANTERIOR AND POSTERIOR
   VENTRICULAR WALLS DURING ACUTE MYOCARDIAL INFARCTION.

7.1. INTRODUCTION

Several studies have demonstrated the utility of
radionuclide ventriculography (RNV) in acute myocardial
infarction (AMI)(1,2,3). A low left ventricular ejection
fraction (LVEF) has prognostic significance as a predictor
of early mortality and the subsequent development of
congestive heart failure or sudden death (4,5,6). The site
of infarction is an important determinant of the outcome of
AMI as well (7). Anterior infarction results in greater LVEF
depression than does inferior infarction (8,9). Right
ventricular infarction is much more common than is generally
appreciated and occurs almost exclusively in patients with
inferior wall infarction (10,11,12). In inferior infarction
the extent of damage and the hemodynamic impact are shared
by both ventricles, whereas the left ventricle bears the
full impact with anterior infarction (9). Invasive as well
as non invasive investigations demonstrated that the
hemodynamic consequence of AMI reflect at least in part the
degree and extent of associated asynergy (13,14).

The purpose of this study was to investigate the
relationship between the evolution of global and regional
ventricular performance during the early phase of AMI. We
used serial EGNA studies to evaluate the effect of infarct

localisation on global LVEF and on the localisation and severity of regional asynergy. Regional asynergy was assessed from amplitude phase functional images after a temporal Fourier transform. By this procedure, the severity of regional wall motion disturbances (RWMD) is not only appreciated in terms of the amplitude of ventricular wall motion but also in terms of abnormalities in the sequence of regional ventricular wall motion (15).

## 7.2. MATERIALS AND METHODS

### 7.2.1. Patient population

81 patients admitted to the coronary care unit with well documented transmural myocardial infarction were studied. The average age of the patients was 60 years (37 to 84). The diagnosis of myocardial infarction was based on the presence of the following criteria : (a) symptoms of chest, arm, neck or back pain suggestive of an acute coronary event, (b) development of pathologic Q waves of more than 0.04 second in duration, (c) serial cardiac enzyme patterns of serum creatine kinase, including its MB isoenzyme fraction, glutamic oxaloacetic transaminase and lactate dehydrogenase that were typical of acute infarction. Patients with a history and/or ECG evidence of prior myocardial infarction or significant valve disease were excluded.

The location of the infarct was characterised as anterior (including anterolateral, anteroseptal or apical infarction or posterolateral infarction) with the use of established electrocardiographic criteria (16). 46 patients were classified as having an anterior infarction, 35 patients as having a posterior infarction.

88

Each patient was assigned on clinical criteria to
Killip classes I-IV upon admission to the CCU (17). 38
patients were in class I, 32 patients were in class II and
11 patients were in class III or IV.

No attempt was made to influence the therapy of
patients involved in this study. All patients were admitted
directly from the emergency room to the CCU. Patients were
treated routinely with bed rest, low flow oxygen by nasal
canula, continuous intravenous lidocain infusion and
heparinisation unless the condition required more vigorous
respiratory or cardiovascular support. 6 patients died
during hospitalisation : 4 had an anterior myocardial
infarction, 2 had a posterior infarction.

## 7.2.2. Radionuclide evaluation

EGNA was performed within 72 hours of hospital
admission in all patients and approximately 10 days (8-12)
after the first study in 75 patients. The technique used for
the data acquisition is described in Chapter 4.2.

Global LVEF was determined from nett time activity
curves generated within a left ventricular region of
interest. The 16 frames of representative cardiac cycle were
corrected for unstructured background by uniform
thresholding, free of operator intervention in a manner
comparable to that described by Goris (18). The threshold
was defined automatically from a cumulative density
distribution function of the end diastolic versus the first
harmonic amplitude of the pixels with a phase corresponding
to ventricular structures. The left ventricular perimeter
was manually traced on a simultaneous display of the first
harmonic amplitude and phase images, the original end
diastolic frame and the background corrected end diastolic

frame. The combined information in those images allows to recognise the maximal extension of the LV area even in severe pathological situations. Nett LV end diastolic and end systolic counts are defined as the maximal and minimal values of the nett LV time/activity curve and the LVEF is determined by the ratio (LVED-LVES)/LVED. To validate the procedure, figure 33 demonstrates the correspondence between 2 successive radionuclide LVEF determinations.

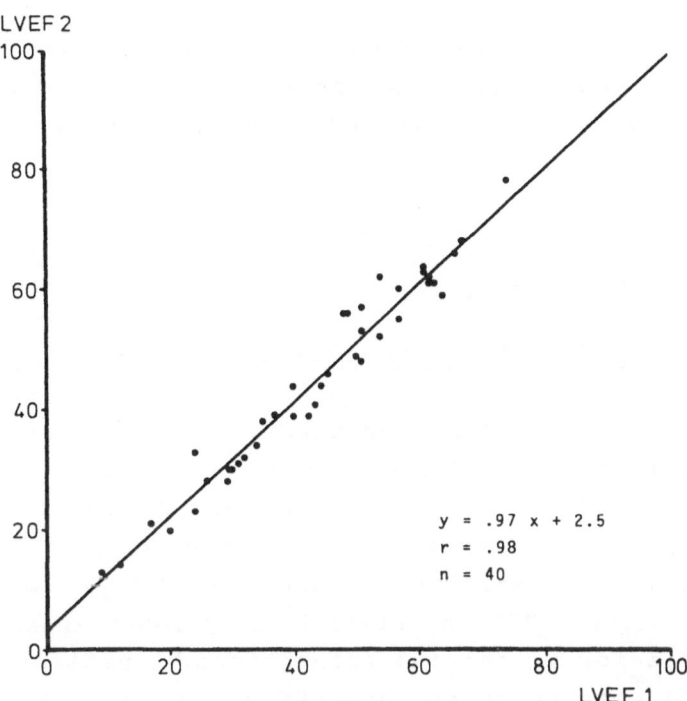

Fig. 33. Reproducibility of LVEF determinations from two successive EGNA studies.

Regional asynergy was evaluated by visual inspection of the first harmonic amplitude and phase functional images, and by amplitude weighted phase distribution histograms of right and left ventricle. RWMD were classified according to their localisation in anterior/anteroseptal (A/AS), apical (AP), posterobasal/posterolateral (PB/PL) or right ventricular (RV) areas, and according to their severity as those with a phase delay of more than or less than 90°.

### 7.2.3. Statistical methods

All data are expressed as mean ± s.d.. The comparison between groups (e.g. anterior vs inferior myocardial infarction) was performed using the Mann Whitney U-test.

### 7.3. RESULTS

### 7.3.1. Global LVEF at the onset of AMI

Global LVEF differed significantly between patients with anterior and with posterior infarction (Table 1, Fig. 34). These differences were observed not only for the whole group, but also when the patients were classified according to Killip classes. Even in the group of patients without complications LVEF was significantly lower in anterior than in posterior myocardial infarctions. 6 patients of Killip class I with anterior infarction had a LVEF below 30, but never exhibited complications during hospitalisation. All the 6 patients who died had severe depressed LVEF: 12-24

Table 1. Global LVEF at the onset of myocardial infarction.

|  | anterior | posterior | statistical significance |
|---|---|---|---|
| Total | 31.5 ± 12.0 | 42.0 ± 13.9 | p < .001 |
| Killip I | 37.2 ± 11.0 | 49.4 ± 9.6 | p < .01 |
| Killip II | 29.6 ± 10.7 | 35.3 ± 12.5 | n.s. |
| Killip III | 17.6 ± 4.6 | 22.8 ± 4.3 | p < .005 |

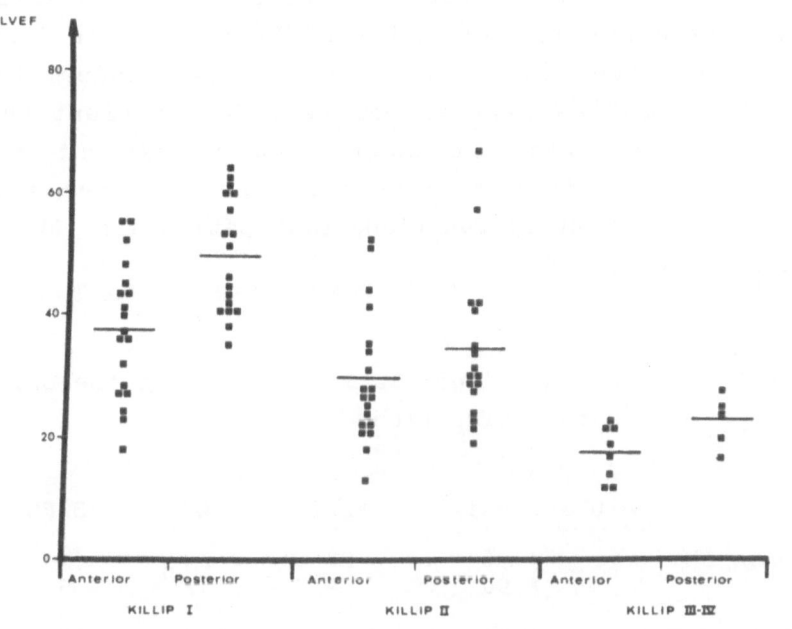

Fig.34. Global LVEF at the onset of myocardial infarction.

## 7.3.2. Identification of infarcted regions by RWMD

Table 2 documents the identification of infarcted regions by the detection of RWMD, the data are further classified according to the observed phase delays.

In the acute phase, 43/46 patients with anterior infarction demonstrated RWMD in the A/AS (36 patients) and/or AP (26 patients) regions. 3 of them showed associated PB/PL anomalies and 1 of them had an associated dyskinesis of the RV apex. In 3/46 patients only minor PB/PL RWMD were evidenced on RNV, the patients had an anterolateral infarction on ECG.

In 28/35 patients with posterior myocardial infarction RWMD were demonstrated in the PB/PL region. In 3 of them there was extension to the antero-apical region, in 13 of them RV anomalies were associated. In 1 patient the only anomaly was localised at the apex and in 4 patients the only LV anomaly was in the AS region, in 2 of them this was associated with RV dysfunction. In 2 patients no RWMD could be evidenced by RNV.

Table 2. Severity and localisation of RWMD at the onset of myocardial infarction.

|  | phase shift | A/AS | AP | PB/PL | RV |
|---|---|---|---|---|---|
| anterior M.I. | < 90 | 27 | 24 | 1 | 1 |
|  | > 90 | 9 | 2 | 5 |  |
| posterior M.I. | < 90 | 3 | 4 | 12 | 13 |
|  | > 90 | 4 |  | 16 | 2 |

No RWMD: 2

The relationship between right ventricular dysfunction and electrocardiographic infarct localisation was more closely investigated. Of the 16 patients with RV wall motion disturbances, 9 had a diaphragmatic infarction, 4 had an inferolateral infarction, 2 had a strictly posteroseptal infarction and only one patient had an anterior infarction.


## 7.3.3. Severity of RWMD

The phase delays observed in PB/PL RWMD were consistently less pronounced than in the other areas. As a result, 34/36 patients with AMI presented phase shifts of more than 90$^\circ$, whereas a similar phase shift of more than 90$^\circ$ was observed in only 14/35 patients with posterior MI.


## 7.3.4. Evolution in global and regional performance

The differences with respect to the abnormalities in regional wall motion became even more pronounced in the radionuclide studies performed 10 days after the onset of M.I. At this moment no RWMD were detectable anymore in 8/35 patients with posterior M.I. The evolution of the regional asynergy in terms of phase alterations for each patients is given in table 3.


Table 3. Evolution of RWMD in anterior and posterior infarctions.

|  | no difference | RWMD | deteriorated RWM |
|---|---|---|---|
| anterior M.I. | 31 | 6 | 9 |
| posterior M.I. | 16 | 15 | 3 |

Figures 35 and 36 represent the evolution in global LVEF, together with their evolution of regional asynchronism in patients with anterior and posterior M.I. respectively.

Only 7/42 patients with anterior M.I. significantly increased their LVEF between the studies performed before 72h and after 10 days. In 31/42 patients, LVEF remained unchanged, in 4/42 patients, LVEF deteriorated further.

The evolution in patients with posterior M.I. was markedly different. In 15/33 patients LVEF increased significantly, no change was observed in 15/33 patients and only 3/33 patients evidenced a decrease in LVEF. Although the 3 patients in which LVEF deteriorated had radionuclide evidence of RV dysfunction, RV involvement in itself did not necessarily determine a limited capacity for improvement, as in other patients with RV involvement, LVEF improved or remained unchanged.

Irrespective of the site of M.I. we observed a good concordance between the evolution in LVEF and the evolution in regional asynchronism.

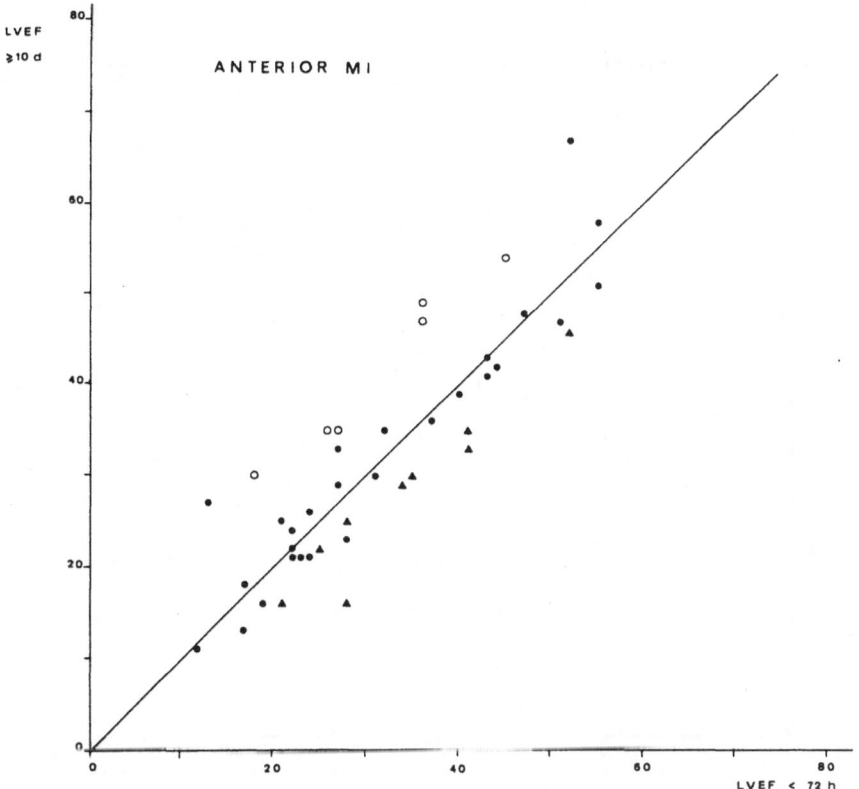

Fig.35. Evolution in LVEF and RWMD in patients with anterior
      myocardial infarction.
         O  ↗ RWMD
         ●  no difference
         ▲  deteriorated RWM

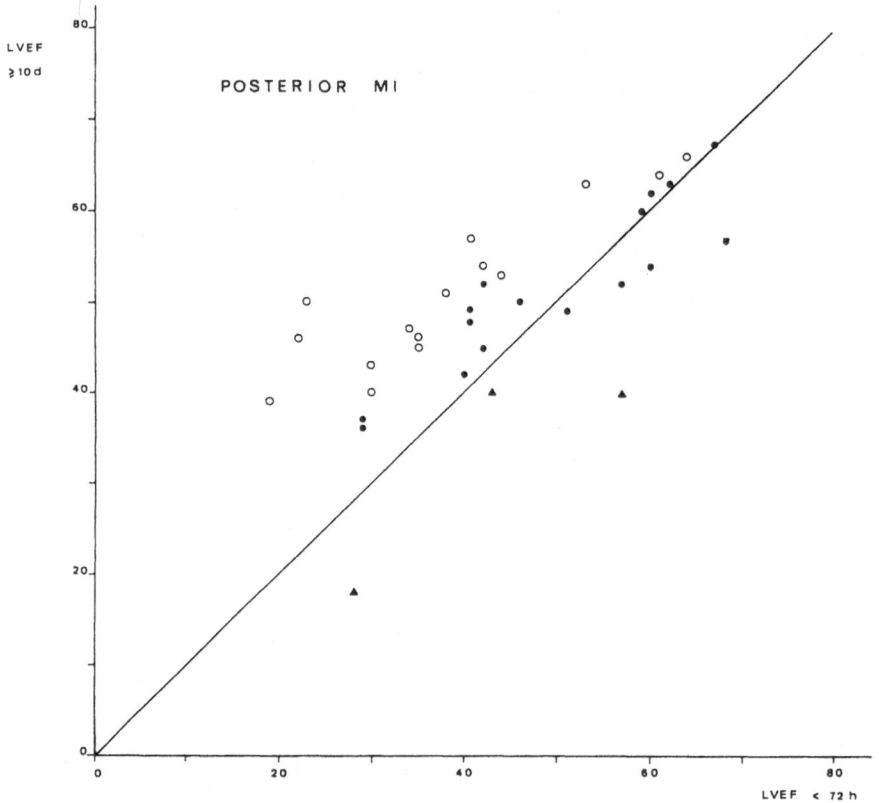

Fig.36. Evolution in LVEF and RWMD in patients with posterior
myocardial infarction.

     O   /   RWMD

     ●   no difference

     ▲   deteriorated RWM

## 7.4. DISCUSSION

Our results thus confirm the data of previous studies which reported a reduced LVEF in patients studied at various times after the onset of AMI and which demonstrated that the site of myocardial infarction may bear importantly on the severity and frequency of depressed LVEF. They further extent these observations in the sense that the differences in LVEF between anterior and posterior myocardial infarction persist, even when the hemodynamic status of the patients, as evaluated clinically, is taken into account. We could also demonstrate a different behaviour of anterior and of posterior M.I. with respect to the early evolution of global and regional ventricular performance. Although these observations should at least in part be attributed to the decrease in sensitivity of RNV for posterior wall disturbances related to absorption phenomena, methodological factors cannot influence the differences observed during the evolution of M.I.

Particular important aspects of this study are the abnormalities in the sequence of wall motion that have been encountered. Alterations in timing of ventricular wall motion are easily investigated by phase analysis of EGNA, while they are not apparent on routine EGNA processed by standard methods, including common functional imaging procedures such as REF or paradox images. The abnormal sequence of LV wall motion may apparently account for alterations in timed ejection fraction (e.g. first third EF).

In this application the evaluation of phase patterns presents several methodological limitations :

1. Visual inspection of functional images remains subjective
2. We only consider a binary distinction between phase delays less or greater than 90°.
3. The sensitivity of amplitude/phase images for the assessment of RWMD is not the same for tangential and non-tangential segments. However, as only modified LAO images were taken into account, the latter factor would in the first place result in an underestimation of the A-AL phase delays.

Notwithstanding these limitation, our study has demonstrated that more severe alterations in the sequence of ventricular wall motion occur with anterior than posterior myocardial infarction. Furthermore, improvement in global response correlated with an improvement in the synchronism of ventricular wall motion. The synchronism of the regional ventricular blood volume changes is a major determinant of intrinsic ventricular pump efficiency. Within the framework of pre- and afterload changes and the Frank Starling mechanisms, differences in the degree of desynchronisation may be expected to result in different adaptations in LVEF and end diastolic volume. Depressed regional ejection fractions in the non-infarcted regions has indeed been observed more frequently in patients with anterior infarction than in patients with posterior infarction (8). These adaptation mechanisms could also explain our observation that for the same Killip classes global LVEF was more severely depressed in anterior than in posterior infarction.

Our study has some practical implications with respect to the interpretation of RNV data. LVEF alone or other indices related to global ventricular volume changes are not sufficient to determine pump function and hemodynamic status in myocardial infarction patients. The functional

dissimilarity of anterior and posterior ventricular walls
emphasises  the need to correlate regional wall motion
response to global ventricular function in a standardised
manner. The amplitude of the regional wall motion is not the
only factor which is thereby involved, and, optimally,
disturbances in the synchronism of ventricular wall motion
should be measured quantitatively.


REFERENCES

1. Rigo P., Murray M., Strauss H.W. et al. 1974. Left
   ventricular function in acute myocardial infarction
   evaluated by gated scintiphotography. Circulation 50,
   678.
2. Schelbert H.R., Henning H., Ashburn W.L. et al. 1976.
   Serial measurements of left ventricular ejection fraction
   by radionuclide angiography early and late after myocardial infarction. Am. J. Cardiol. 38, 405.
3. Reduto L.A, Berger H.J., Cohen Z.S. et al. 1978. Sequential radionuclide assessment of right ventricular performance after acute transmural myocardial infarction.
   Ann. Intern. Med. 89, 441.
4. Taylor G. J., Huphries J.O., Mellitis E.D. et al. 1980.
   Predictors of clinical course, coronary anatomy and left
   ventricular function after recovery from acute myocardial infarction. Circulation 62, 960.
5. Battler A., Slutsky R., Karliner J. et al. 1980. Left
   ventricular ejection fraction and first third ejection
   fraction early after acute myocardial infarction: value
   for predicting mortality and morbidity. Am. J. Cardiol.
   45, 197.
6. Shah P.K., Pichler M., Berman D.S. et al.1980. Left ventricular ejection fraction and first third ejection
   fraction determined by radionuclide ventriculography in
   early stages of first transmural myocardial infarction:
   relation to short term prognosis. Am. J. Cardiol. 45,
   542.
7. Bulkley B.H. 1981. Site and sequelae of myocardial
   infarction. New Eng. J. Med. 6, 337.
8. Wynne L.M., Sayers M., Maddox D.E., et al. 1980. Regional left ventricular function in acute myocardial
   infarction: evaluation with quantitative ventriculography. Am. J. Cardiol. 45, 203.
9. Marmor A., Geltman, Biello D.R., et al. 1981.
   Function response of the right ventricle to myocardial
   infarction: dependence on the site of left ventricular
   infarction. Circulation 64, 1005.

10. Rigo P., Murray M., Taylor D.R., et al. 1975. Right ventricular dysfunction detected by gated scintigraphy in patients with acute inferior myocardial infarction. Circulation 52, 268.
11. Tobinick E., Schelbert H.R., Henning H., et al. 1978. Right ventricular ejection fraction in patients with acute anterior and inferior myocardial infarction assessed by radionuclide angiography. Circulation 57, 1078.
12. Walton S.,Rowlands D.J., Shields R.A. et al. 1979. Study of right ventricular function in ischemic heart disease using radionucide angiocardiography. Intensive Care med. 53, 121.
13. Bertrand M.E., Rousseau J.M., Lablanche J.M. et al. 1979. Cineangiographic assessment of left ventricular function in the acute phase of transmural myocardial infarction. Am. J. Cardiol. 43, 472.
14. Rigaud M., Rocha P., Boschat J. et al. 1979. Regional left ventricular function assessed by contrast angiography in acute myocardial infarction. Circulation. 60, 130.
15. Bossuyt A., Huyghens L., Deconinck F. et al. 1982. Relationship between global and regional ventricular performance during acute myocardial infarction studied by amplitude/ phase analysis. In: Nuclear Medicine and Biology Raynaud C. (Ed.) II, 1813.
16. Winsor T. 1968. Principles of electrocardiography in myocardial infarction. In: The Ciba Collection Heart Netter F. (Ed.) Vol 5.
17. Killip T., Kimball J.T. 1967. Treatment of myocardial infarction in a coronary care unit. A two years experience with 250 patients. Am. J. Cardiol. 20, 457.
18. Goris M.L., Briandet P.A., Huffer E. 1979. Automation and operator independent data processing of cardiac and pulmonary functions: role, methods and results. In: Information Processing in Medical Imaging. Di Paola R. (Ed.) INSERM 88, 427.

8. SCINTIGRAPHIC VISUALISATION OF THE EFFECT OF CONDUCTION DISTURBANCES ON THE MECHANICAL EVENTS OF THE CARDIAC CYCLE.

8.1. INTRODUCTION

In the presence of ventricular conduction disturbances, activation of the ventricles is no longer synchronous (1). Muscular contraction is expected to be correspondingly asynchronous. However, disturbances in ventricular contraction resulting from abnormal electrical activation are difficult to demonstrate hemodynamically because of the complexity of these events and the rapidity with which they occur (2). Equilibrium gated cardiac blood pool scintigraphy allows the simultaneous study of the volume changes occuring in both ventricles during an averaged cardiac cycle. Alterations in the time sequence of these volume changes, as they are displayed by the phase image, should allow to visualise the alterations in the mechanical events of the cardiac cycle resulting from electrophysiological disturbances of the heart, such as bundle branch blocks or pace maker stimulation (3,4).

8.2. BUNDLE BRANCH BLOCKS

In this study, the synchronism in the blood volume changes between and within the right and left ventricles was evaluated by means of the first harmonic amplitude/phase patterns displayed in the functional images and in the amplitude/phase distribution histograms of each of the ventricles taken separately (5).

The study group consisted of 42 patients. As defined by ECG at the time of the study, 9 patients presented a complete RBBB, 17 patients a complete LBBB and 13 patients had signs of left anterior hemiblock (LAH). Only patients with regular cardiac rhythm were studied. Concomittant cardiovascular disease was present in most of these patients but 9 patients (4 RBBB - 5 LBBB) were asymptomatic and presented no other signs of cardiovascular abnormalities.

A typical amplitude/phase distribution pattern was present in patients with LBBB, RBBB, but not in patients with hemiblocks. All LBBB patterns were characterised by a bimodal amplitude/phase distribution over both ventricles taken together. The difference between the mean phase of the left and right ventricles ranged between 27° and 60° (Fig.37), which is significantly different from the findings in normal individuals where, within statistical limits, the phases in both ventricles are identical. The earliest phase was in the septal region spreading first over the right ventricle and thereafter over the left ventricle (Fig. 38).

In patients with a RBBB, the amplitude/phase histogram was also bimodal, the difference between the mean phase of both ventricles ranging from 18° to 48°.The earliest phase was in the left ventricle and spreads via the apex to the right ventricle.

In the absence of associated regional wall motion disturbances, the aspect of the amplitude image was normal in BBB patients. To some extent, phase shifts in localised asynergic areas can distinctly be recognised from the BBB patients if the additional information of the amplitude of the corresponding count rate changes is taken into account. As illustrated in Figure 39, superimposed on the LBBB pattern, we can recognise a dyskinetic movement of the left ventricular apex as a region with markedly decreased amplitude and a phase shift of more than 90°.

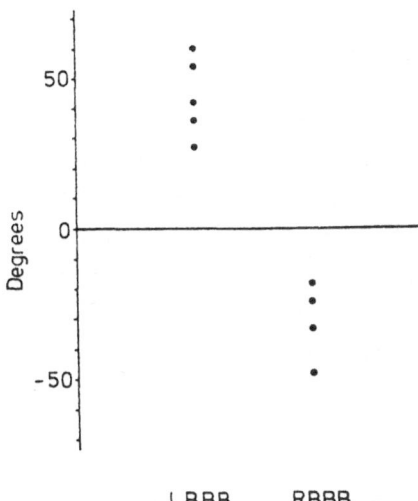

Fig.37. Comparison of differences of mean phases in left and right ventricle (LV-RV) in patients with LBBB and RBBB without known concomittant cardiovascular disease.

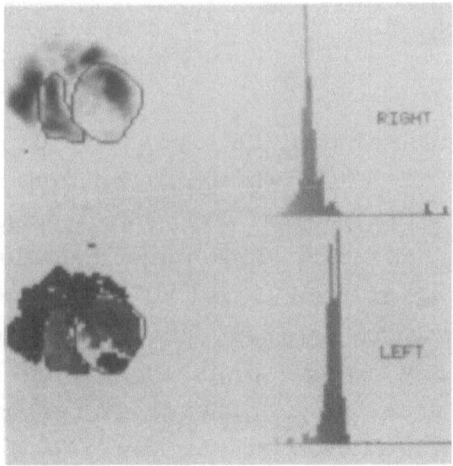

Fig.39. Anteroseptal dyskinesis superimposed on LBBB pattern in a patient with a myocardial infarction.

## 8.3. EFFECT OF VARIOUS KINDS OF PACE MAKER STIMULATION AND PACING FREQUENCIES ON VENTRICULAR PUMP FUNCTION

### 8.3.1. Introduction

While modern programmable pace makers allow for a noninvasive selection of a wide range of pacing modes and pacing rates, the hemodynamic effects of pace maker treatment are often difficult to prove. In this study, we investigated by temporal Fourier transform the movements of the blood pool as they are affected by the mode and frequency of pace maker stimulation.

### 8.3.2. Methodology

A group of 18 patients with multiprogrammable pace maker units were studied. Mean age was 70 years. 9 patients presented a cardiomyopathy, in most of the cases due to ischemic heart disease or hypertension. 9 patients had no cardiomyopathy. The presence or absence of cardiomyopathy was assessed on clinical grounds : complaints and physical signs, chest X-ray and the need for diuretic and cardiotonic drugs.

RNV was performed at rest at different pacing frequencies (80-100-120 beats/min.) and on different pacing modes (AV sequential pacing (DVI) and ventricular inhibited (VVI)). Whenever possible, data were recorded after 5 to 10 minutes of pacing at each level of frequency. Hemodynamic data were obtained in the same conditions for evaluation of pulmonary artery wedge pressure (PAWP) and pressure morphology. The presence or absence of retrograde P waves in VVI stimulation was looked for on ECG and the pressure curve.

8.3.3. <u>Results</u>

Figure 40 illustrates the effect of pace maker stimulation in one of the patients studied twice : in normal sinus rhythm and with pacemaker stimulation at a rate of 70/min. The site of pace maker stimulation can clearly be recognised by the early phase in the right ventricular apex. The phase first spreads over the right ventricle and then over the left ventricle, resulting in a bimodal amplitude/phase distribution between both ventricles. The shape and spread of the amplitude/phase histogram within the ventricles is also disturbed, pace maker stimulation markedly increasing the spread of the left ventricular phases. On the functional images, we observe a phase shift between the infero-apical region and the lateral border of the left ventricle, indicating that the mechanical contraction starts at the site of pace maker stimulation and then progresses to the rest of the ventricles. As at least part of conduction proceeds via ventricular muscle rather than via the His Purkinje system, the progression of the phases in the left ventricle is slow.

Ventricular pacing (DVI or VVI) at high frequencies (100 - 120/min.) produced desynchronisation within the left ventricle always located in the same area : inferoseptal and apical (Fig. 41). This may occur even in patients with normal coronary angiogram and is thus probably independent of the presence of CAD. The degree of desynchronisation was more pronounced in patients with cardiomyopathy. Concomittant with this desynchronisation, we observed a fall in ejection fraction and an increase in end diastolic volume in these patients. When present, the phase shifts observed in an individual patient were more important at V 120 pacing rates than at V 100. This difference still persisted when the phase values were converted in their equivalent in msec. This indicates that the desynchronisation cannot solely be explained by a slow conduction rate and delayed ventricular activation, but that disturbances in myocardial contraction and relaxation are probably interrelated.

Retrograde ventriculo-atrial conduction during VVI pacing was observed in 10 patients. Whereas in VVI pacing with AV dissociation or atrial fibrillation, atrial volume changes occured independently of the ventricles, in VVI pacing with retrograde atrial activation, volume changes in the right atrium occured nearly in phase with the lateral wall of the left ventricle (Fig.42). In these patients, sequential related volume changes are observed on the phase images in DVI pacing. Switching from DVI to VVI pacing in this subgroup produces a fall in cardiac output, an increase in PAPW and a giant retrograde A wave. While we observed a fall in the ejection fraction of the patients with cardiomyopathy, the patients without cardiomyopathy were able to increase their ejection fraction, but only at basal heart rate.

## 8.3.4. Comments

Ventriculo-atrial conduction has been identified as a key risk factor for ventricular pace maker syndrome. As atrial contraction occurs within the ventricular ejection period, blood is pumped backwards into the pulmonary and systemic venous beds. Retrograde P waves on the surface ECG may not be detected because of baseline abnormalities or low voltage. Amplitude/phase functional mapping of EGNA may non-invasively elucidate the pathophysiological mechanisms in such circumstances.

In those patients where ventricular pacing at higher frequencies induces a desynchronisation of the volume changes within the left ventricular, the higher pacing rates from the apex of the right ventricle, as now available with physiological pacing, could have deleterious effects.

## 8.4. DISCUSSION

This study illustrates how strongly parametric imaging may improve the visualisation of time patterns in scintigraphic studies, The distinct phase patterns that were identified for various intraventricular conduction disturbances correlate with electrophysiological findings. In each case the phase image seemed to correspond to currently held concepts of activation sequence for the above conditions. The phase itself however cannot be considered as an electrical activation map. Indeed, radionuclide ventriculography studies the volume changes in the cardiac chambers during a heart cycle. Alterations in the time sequence of these volume changes as displayed by the phase image could result from alterations in electrical activation, myocardial contraction and relaxation, blood ejection or passive movements. Furthermore, the temporal Fourier transform used here was limited to the evaluation of the volume changes at the fundamental frequency. Changes in the symmetry between systolic and diastolic events will affect the fitting of the first harmonic to the real time/activity curves.

The use of a cinematic display of the onset of mechanical systole was introduced by Verba (6) to obtain information similar to that of the phase image. With this method, the total Fourier transform of each pixel is calculated and multiplied by a filter function. The second derivate of the inverse transform is then used to determine the point in the cardiac cycle at which emptying started for each pixel. The whole procedure requires a large computer or the incorporation of array processors to nuclear medicine computer systems (7) to perform the operation within acceptable time limits. It should furthermore be emphasised that, whatever calculation algorithm or display procedure is used, the accuracy of the method is determined by the filter in the frequency domain. The latter approach allows the functional imaging of ventricular emptying and filling taken separately.

Notwithstanding the limitation to the first harmonic model, the amplitude and phase images allow the characterisation of typical contraction patterns in different types of intraventricular conduction disturbances. Since 1980 similar observations have been repeatedly reported by several groups of investigators who also demonstrated abnormal phase patterns in patients with sustained ventricular tachycardia and with Wolf Parkinson White syndrome (8,9,10,11).

From a clinical point of view, the recognition of distinct amplitude/phase patterns related to disturbances in electrical activation appears to be especially useful for the localisation of myocardial infarction in patients with BBB and as an aid to determine the optimal site and frequency for pace maker stimulation.

## REFERENCES

1.  Van Dam R. Th. 1976. Ventricular activation in human and canine bundle branch block. In: The conduction system of the heart. Wellens H.J., Lie K.I. Janse M.J. (Eds.) 377.
2.  Braunwald E., Morrow A. 1957. Sequence of ventricular contraction in human bundle branch block. Am. J. Med. 23, 205.
3.  Deconinck F., Bossuyt A., Lepoudre R. 1979. Regional ventricular wall motion assessed by temporal Fourier transform. Proc. 4th Annual Western Regional Meeting, Soc. Nucl. Med.
4.  Bossuyt A., Deconick F., Lepoudre R. 1980. Application d'une échelle de couleurs cyclique, élément essentiel dans l'étude fonctionnelle de phénomènes périodiques. Int. J. Med. & Biol. 7, 231.
5.  Bossuyt A., Deconinck F. 1981. Scintigraphic visualisation of the effect of conduction disturbances on the mechanical events of the cardiac cycle. Annals World Ass. Med. Inform. 1, 1.

6.  Verba J., Bornstein I., Alazraki N.P. et al. 1979. Onset
    and progression of mechanical systole derived from gated
    radionuclide techniques and displayed in cine format. J.
    Nucl. Med. 20, 625.
7.  King M.A., Doherty P.W. 1982. Cardiac image processing
    using an array processor. In: Digital Imaging Clinical
    Advances in Nuclear Medicine. Esser P. (Ed.) 153.
8.  Pavel D., Byrom E., Swiryn S. et al. Normal and abnormal
    electrical activation of the heart: Imaging patterns
    obtained by phase analysis of equilibrium cardiac stu-
    dies. In Medical Radionuclide Imaging II. IAEA-SM-247,
    253.
9.  Links J., Douglas K.H., Wagner H.N. 1980. Patterns of
    ventricular emptying by Fourier analysis of gated blood
    pool studies. J. Nucl. Med. 21, 978.
10. Swiryn S., Pavel D., Byrom E. et al. 1981. Sequential
    regional phase mapping of radionuclide gated biventricu-
    lograms in patients with left bundle branch block. Am.
    Heart J. 102, 1000.
11. Adam W.E., Sigel H., Zaorska-Rajca J. et al. 1983.
    Utility of Imaging Techniques to Predict and Manage
    Patients with Cardiovscular Abnormalities. In: Diagnstic
    Imaging in Medicine. Reba R., Goodenough D., Davidson H.
    (Eds.) 452.

9. PARAMETRIC IMAGING AND TEMPORAL CONTRAST ENHANCEMENT FOR
   THE VISUALISATION OF TIME PATTERNS.

9.1. DATA COMPRESSION THROUGH EFFICIENT DATA ACQUISITION AND
     PROCESSING

9.1.1. The Hadamard transform

The use off the Fourier transform limited to the first
harmonic for functional imaging in equilibrium gated nuclear
angiography (EGNA) does not provide an exact description of
the time function. The Fourier transform is used to extract
parameters which give a clinically adequate description of
the activity changes in each pixel : first harmonic
amplitude $A_1$ and phase $\phi_1$. Higher harmonic parameters as
such may be of interest, but their clinical significance has
not been clearly demonstrated yet.

The Fourier transform is based on multiplications of
the functions to be transformed by sine and cosine
functions.

Let $I(t)$ be the function to be transformed.

$$I(t) = A_0 + B_1 \sin \omega t + C_1 \cos \omega t$$
$$+ B_2 \sin 2\omega t + C_2 \cos 2\omega t$$
$$+ \text{higher harmonics}$$

In the case of functional imaging, where $I(t) = I_1, \ldots, I_i, \ldots, I_n$ is the original transformed image series,

$$B_j = \frac{2}{n} \sum_{i=1}^{n} I_i \ \sin \{j \frac{2\pi}{n} (i-1)\}$$

$$C_j = \frac{2}{n} \sum_{i=1}^{n} I_i \ \cos \{j \frac{2\pi}{n} (i-1)\}$$

The Fourier transform is computationally difficult to perform on a real time basis during data acquisition. We therefore investigated the use of a square wave basis function to calculate parametric images. The square wave function which we use is shown in Figure 43 and varies from +1 to -1. Two periods are shown, but the information is periodic from x = - ∞ to + ∞ When the origin of the X-axis intercepts the function in point S, the wave function is y = SQSN (x) (square sine). When the origin is at C, the function is y = SQCN (x) (square cosine).

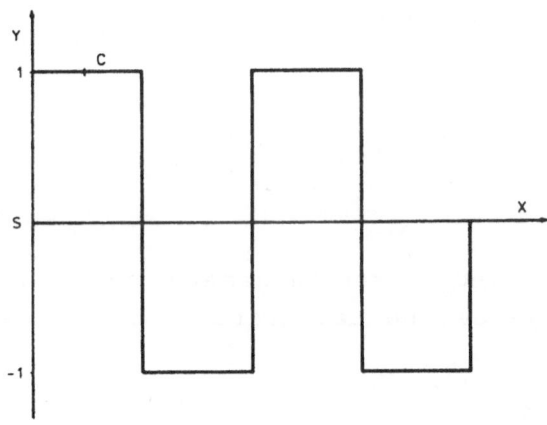

Fig. 43 Square wave function.

The use of square wave functions for the linear transformation of functions is a Hadamard or Walsh transform (1). The square wave function itself can be analysed in terms of a Fourier·series.

$$SQSN\ (x)\ =\ \frac{4}{\pi}\ (\sin\ (x)\ +\ \frac{1}{3}\sin\ (3x)\ +\ \frac{1}{5}\sin\ (5x)\ +\ ...\ )$$

$$SQCN\ (x)\ =\ \frac{4}{\pi}\ (\cos\ (x)\ -\ \frac{1}{3}\cos\ (3x)\ +\ \frac{1}{5}\cos\ (5x)\ -\ ...\ )$$

Substitution yields (the constant scaling factors have been deleted for simplification) :

$$B_1\ =\ \sum_{i=1}^{n}\ I_1\ SQSN\ (\frac{2\pi}{n}\ (i\ -\ 1))$$

$$=\ \sum_{i=1}^{n}\ I_1\ \sin\ (\frac{2\pi}{n}\ (i\ -\ 1))$$

$$+\ \frac{1}{3}\ \sum_{i=1}^{n}\ I_1\ \sin\ (\frac{2\pi.3}{n}\ (i\ -\ 1))$$

$$+\ \frac{1}{5}\ \sum_{i=1}^{n}\ I_1\ \sin\ (\frac{2\pi.5}{n}\ (i\ -\ 1))$$

$$+\ ...$$

$$=\ B_1\ +\ \frac{1}{3}B_3\ +\ \frac{1}{5}B_5\ +\ ...$$

and

$$C_1\ =\ C_1\ -\ \frac{1}{3}C_3\ +\ \frac{1}{5}C_5\ +\ ...$$

By means of $B_1$ and $C_1$ the "Hadamard" first harmonic amplitude and phase can be calculated and displayed as parametric images .

$$A\ =\ (B_1^2\ +\ C_1^2)^{1/2}$$

$$\phi\ =\ arctg\ (-\ B/C)$$

When the image series consists of a multiple of four images, the Hadamard transform reduces the image series to four images $I_1$, $I_2$, $I_3$ and $I_4$, each spanning one fourth of the total acquisition length. By means of four images, the Hadamard first harmonic amplitude A and phase $\phi$ can be calculated as follows :

$$A = \{(I_1 + I_2 - I_3 - I_4)^2 + (I_1 - I_2 - I_3 + I_4)^2\}^{1/2}$$

$$\phi = \text{arctg} \left(- \frac{I_1 + I_2 - I_3 - I_4}{I_1 - I_2 - I_3 + I_4}\right)$$

## 9.1.2. The comparison of the Fourier and Hadamard transform in EGNA.

The Fourier and Hadamard amplitude or phase are not equal when the original image series contains more than four images (there is no 2nd or higher harmonic when the sampling frequency is limited to 4 images/cycle). When there is a multiple of four images, the Hadamard transform reduces the image series to 4 images before transforming them. When there are four images, the Hadamard and Fourier transform differ only by constants.

In EGNA, it is usual to acquire at least 16 images per cycle. The Fourier and Hadamard first harmonic amplitude and phase will be equivalent if the information content of the 3rd and higher odd harmonics is negligible as compared with the information content of the first harmonic. The information content of different harmonics will not be the same for all pixels. Within heart structures, the first harmonic Fourier component of the time activity curves (TAC) is by far more important than the contribution of the 3rd or higher harmonics. The Hadamard transform filters, the higher harmonics by means of the scaling factors 1/3, 1/5,..., so that their contribution to the functional images is negligible. As a result, the use of the Hadamard transform demonstrates that four images/cycle, which each span one fourth cycle, yield high phase and amplitude resolution functional images in EGNA (Fig.44). With an acquisition memory size limited to 64 kbyte, one now has the option to acquire 4 high resolution 128 x 128 images per cycle. This allows the gated acquisition of seven-pinhole images for tomographic imaging (2).

Figure 45 shows an example provided by EGNA of the equivalence between Fourier functional phase imaging and Hadamard functional imaging using 16 images/cycle.

## 9.2. TEMPORAL CONTRAST ENHANCEMENT

By discarding the information contained in the higher harmonics, all information regarding possible asymmetry in the pixel's TAC is lost in first harmonic amplitude/phase imaging. To illustrate this effect wecompared the' first harmonic amplitude/phase patterns with regional TAC in selected case studies of patients with various kinds of valvular heart disease.

Valve dysfunction results in disturbances in ventricular blood volume changes by multiple underlying mechanisms : alterations in myocardial contraction and relaxation consecutive to myocardial hypertrophy and volume overload. Each of these factors can influence the ultimate amplitude/phase pattern, but introduces a lack of specificity of the functional images for a given pathological process.

Figure 46 represents the radionuclide data of a patients with aortic stenosis. The amplitude/phase histograms and the functional images show a bimodal distribution of the phases in both ventricles comparable to that observed in patients with left bundle branch block. By comparing the TAC in both ventricles, it can be concluded that the phase delay corresponds to a prolonged LV ejection time, which was confirmed by the clinical observation.

Figure 47 represents a similar radionuclide observation in a patient with a mitral valve prothesis. The time/activity patterns are comparable in aspect to these observed in the previous example. But from the TAC it is now obvious that the major disturbances occur during LV filling.

In both instances the shape of the right and left ventricular TAC is best compared when their display is

scaled : the scaling in figure 47 equalises the minimum value
of the two curves as well as their maximum value. This
eliminates all information on the magnitude of the activity
changes and displays only the timing information.

We propose a temporal contrast enhancement procedure
which implements on a pixel by pixel basis the scaling of
the TAC to their minimum value (3). In the image series, the
number of photons in each pixel (x,y) varies as a function
of time : N(t) represents the individual pixel TAC. Each
pixel TAC will reach a minimum value Nmin in the series. The
function N(t) can now be decomposed as N(t) = Nmin + N'(t).
Nmin does not depend on t and N'(t) becomes zero in at least
one image of the series. For each pixel a value Nmin can be
determined and all the values can be stored in a "minimum"
image. In this image each pixel corresponds to the minimum
ever reached by all the corresponding pixels of the image
series along the temporal axis. When a percentage of this
image is substracted from the original series, a
corresponding percentage in temporal contrast enhancement is
achieved. In the limit of 100 % substraction, the temporal
contrast enhancement is maximal, as for each pixel there is
at least one image of the processed series in which the
activity in the pixel will become zero. The image series
displays magnitude and temporal information.

By normalising the series for magnitude changes
(dividing the series by its "maximum" images) to 100, a
series representing temporal information only is obtained.
Freeman (4) has called this latter procedure fractional
variation imaging. The methods provide a very powerful means
for improving the interpretation of the study by visualising
temporal changes in activity that were not perceptible due
to their low temporal contrast. (Fig. 48.)

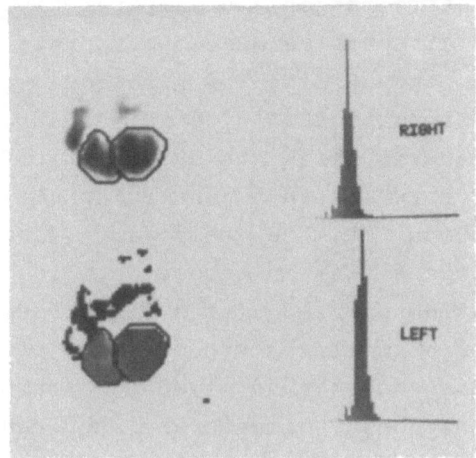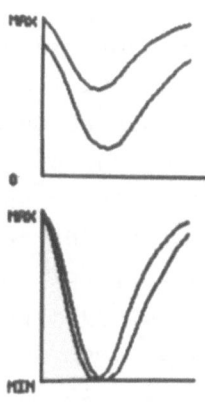

Fig. 46. Aortic stenosis.

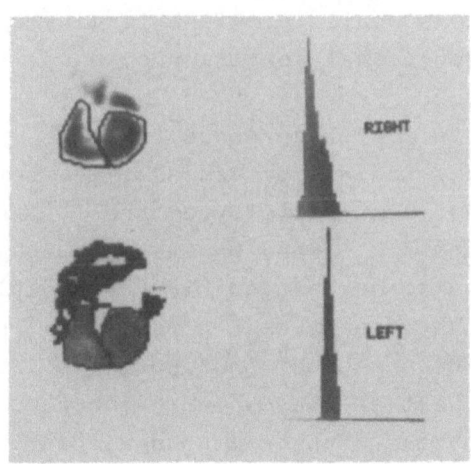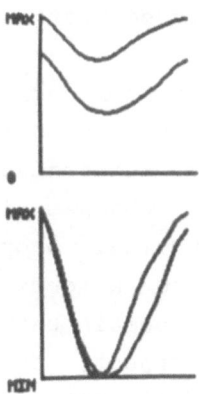

Fig. 47. Mitral valve prosthesis.

## 9.3. DISCUSSION

Amplitude/phase parametric images and temporal contrast enhancement represent two alternative means to improve the perception of magnitude and timing of motion. Both procedures optimise the information density in the data set according to particular criteria which are choosen to favor information which is most relevant in a particular clinical situation. The application of the temporal Hadamard transform to EGNA demonstrates that in those applications where the temporal information carried by the first harmonic is satisfactory, parametric imaging overcomes some of the limitations due to photon noise and limited temporal sampling. It is shown that only 4 images are required to calculate clinically relevant first harmonic amplitude and phase on a pixel by pixel basis. When only three images per cycle are used, the integration of the information during one-third of the cycle mixes the first and higher harmonic information such that the 16 image and 3 image first harmonic functional images are no longer equivalent. The temporal Hadamard transform provides efficient and relevant data compression and allows smaller digital imaging systems to handle sophisticated functional imaging procedures (2).

Pattern recognition in amplitude/phase imaging assumes a temporal model for the studied processed. By temporal contrast enhancement the detectability of the timing of activity changes is improved, based on the knowledge of psychophysical properties of our vision (5). Rose (6) has introduced a formalism that describes the relation in the spatial domain between the number of photons in the images of an object, the contrast of the object, the number of spatial elements (pixels) that can be distinguished in the image and the statistical confidence with which we can distinguish this number of elements. He has shown that the number of elements that can be distinguished is proportional to the square of the contrast. His approach emphasises the effect of contrast and photon statistics in medical imaging (7). Weber's law states that the just noticeable difference in light intensity I between two pixels is a linear function of the average intensity of the pixel itself: $\Delta I/I = $ cte (8). Kelly has shown that the just noticeable difference $\Delta I$ of intensity variations in time of an image with average intensity I is also a function of the temporal frequency at which the variation occurs. The differences in timing of changes in intensity in different parts of an image are extremely difficult to evaluate when the changes are just noticeable or when the changes are superimposed on a large steady intensity. Kelly's experiments have a demonstrated a property of our vision which limits strongly our perception of useful information in movie displays of dynamic isotope studies : our eye is much more sensitive to small variations in intensity at 10-20 Hz than at 1 Hz. We tend to look at heart studies at a "natural" frequency of 1 Hz. At this frequency the individual image noise varies at the frequency for which we are most sensitive. This is one of the reasons why temporal smoothing can improve a movie display.

Rose's formalism, Weber's law and Kelly's experiments suggest temporal contrast enhancement to improve the perception of time patterns.

In terms of a temporal Fourier analysis the contrast enhanced series of images contains all the Fourier frequencies except the zero frequency component. As the method is based on the substraction of a constant image, the count rate changes in the processed series are still linearly related to the changes in blood volume but all information about absolute ventricular volume is lost.

REFERENCES

1. Pratt W.K. 1978. Digital Image Pocessing. Wiley-Inter-science Publications (Eds.) 250.
2. Deconinck F., Bossuyt A., Lepoudre R. 1982. Temporal contrast enhancement and parametric imaging for the visualisation of time patterns in dynamic scintigraphic imaging. Nuklearmedizin Suppl. 20, 25.
3. Deconinck F., Bossuyt A., Lepoudre R. 1982. New approaches for the analysis and visualisation of time patterns in dynamic scintigraphic imaging. Nuclear Medicine and Biology I. Raynaud C. (Ed.) 39.
4. Freeman M.L., Barnes W.E., Gose E.E. 1982. Application of time-domain analysis to gated cardiac blood-pool studies. In: Digital Imaging Clinical Advances in Nuclear Medicine. Esser P. (Ed.) 217.
5. Deconinck F., Bossuyt A., Lepoudre R. 1981. The visualisation of time patterns in dynamic scintigraphic imaging. IEEE Visual Psychophysics and Medical Imaging. 43.
6. Rose A. 1973. Vision - Human and electronic. Plenum Press N.Y.
7. Shosa D., Kaufmann L. 1981. Methods for evaluation of diagnostic imaging instrumentation. Phys. Med. Biol. 26. 101.
8. Cornsweet T.N. 1970. Visual Perception. Academic Press New York.

# 10. RADIONUCLIDE INDICES OF CARDIAC FUNCTION RELATED TO STRUCTURAL VENTRICULAR DISORDERS

## 10.1. INTRODUCTION

The purpose of this study is to define indices of cardiac function which should allow a quantification of structural ventricular disturbances, such as regional wall motion disturbances (RWMD), in terms of magnitude and timing of regional volume changes (1,2).

Parametric images of the first harmonic amplitude and phase of the volume changes have proven their clinical applicability for the evaluation of RWMD and for the visualisation of the hemodynamic effect of disturbances in electrical activation. The chief limitation of visual assessment of amplitude/phase images is its subjectivity. Statistical analysis of phase distribution is currently under investigation as an objective technique for detecting the presence and/or severity of RWMD (3,4,5). A binary decision whether RWM is normal or abnormal may probably be achieved by analysis of amplitude weighted phase distribution functions or by evaluation of the clustering properties of the amplitude/phase distribution in the complex plane (6). Obtaining a set of quantitative indices should however be the goal of a diagnostic measuring technique performed at rest and during physiologic or therapeutic interventions. With respect to this, amplitude/phase imaging is hampered by the fact that only the basic frequency component of the activity changes is analysed (7).

In this study we quantified regional ventricular function in terms of magnitude and timing of motion by means of parameters which take into account all the Fourier frequencies of an averaged cardiac cycle except the zero frequency component (which bears no dynamic information).

## 10.2. MATERIALS AND METHODS

### 10.2.1. Definition of the indices.

Using the original (preprocessed) data of an EGNA study, a time/activity curve is calculated for each pixel. Two images representing the minima and the maxima of each pixel's time/activity curve are reconstructed (MAX image, MIN image). The original images representing the activity distribution at end diastole and at end systole are used as such (ED image, ES image). Within a region of interest (ROI) over the left ventricle the counts in MAX, MIN, ED and ES images are calculated. We define:

$$CI = \frac{ED-ES}{ED-MIN}$$

$$FI = \frac{ED-ES}{MAX-ES}$$

$$EFF = \frac{ED-ES}{MAX-MIN}$$

Figure 49 illustrates how asynchronism and magnitude of count rate changes will affect the parameters defined in this way. Three ROI are considered. They are choosen so that ROI1 = ROI2 + ROI3, and that the count rate changes inside both ROI2 and ROI3 occur synchronously. The upper figures represent the time activity curves in ROI2 and ROI3. The figures beneath represent the resultant time activity curve (ROI1). As illustrated in (A) all indices in ROI1 will reach 100% as soon as, and only if the count rate changes between ROI2 and ROI3 occur synchronously. CI and Eff will decrease as soon as the time at which ROI2 and ROI3 reach a minimum value is different (B). FI and Eff will decrease as soon as the time at which ROI2 and ROI3 reach a maximum value is different (C). (D) shows a general situation whereby magnitude and timing of the count rate changes are different for ROI2 and ROI3.

Thus, CI and FI respectively describe the synchronicity at which the left ventricle arrives at a minimum or at a maximum. A decrease in CI and FI will only be identical when the alterations related to the timing of emptying and the timing of filling are symmetrical. ED-ES corresponds to the real stroke volume. MAX-MIN corresponds to the sum of all the Fourier amplitudes excepted the zero frequency. As such, Eff can be considered as the ratio of the effective volume changes to the total volume changes which occur as a result of asynchronism in myocardial wall motion.

124

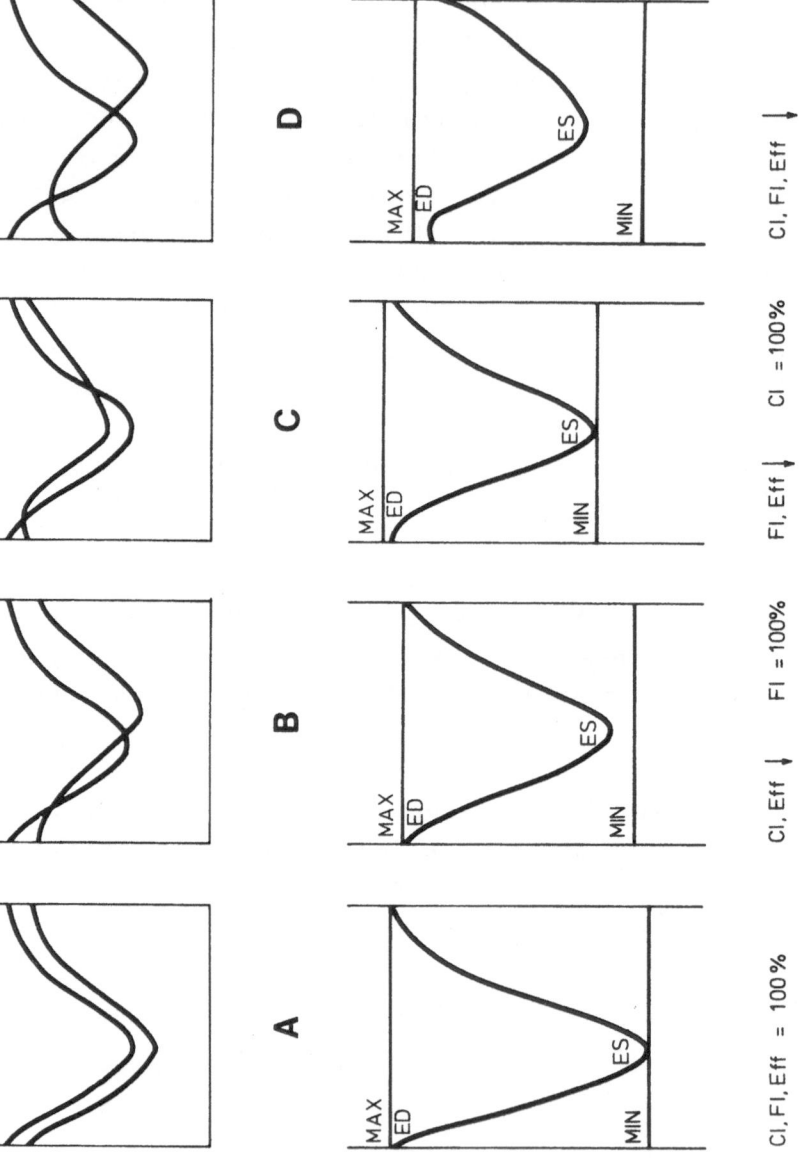

Fig.49. Effect of regional asynchronism on indices.

## 10.2.2. Effect of noise

As MAX and MIN values are calculated by a counting process on a pixel by pixel basis their measurement is subject to large systematic errors induced by statistical noise. The probability of overestimating the time maximum on a noisy TAC is greater than the probability to underestimate it. When all measured maxima are added to determine MAX, there is a great probability of obtaining an overestimation of the real value. Similarly, there exists a fairly great probability to underestimate MIN. In contrast the error in the determination of ED and ES is much smaller: these values do not result from a summation of parameters obtained on pixel TACs with low counting statistics, but are defined on global LVTAC with much higher counting statistics.

Experimentally, the sensitivity of the indices to statistical noise was investigated in 5 patients who had 4 consecutive EGNA studies. The data acquisition periods were so that 1 *, 2 *, 4 * and 8 * $10^6$ counts were obtained in the total field of view. The position of the patient did not change between the 4 data acquisition periods. The LV ROI was delineated manually on the amplitude, phase and end diastolic images derived from the 8 * $10^6$ counts series. For each of the 4 image series LVEFF calculated in this ROI was plotted against the total number of counts in the study (Fig.50). EFF appears to increase as the counting statistics increase. Above a certain threshold, the curves are found to become parallel, indicating a common systematic error affecting the different clinical situations. As depicted in figure 51, preprocessing of the raw data ( temporal filtering with kernel 121 followed by spatial 9 point convolution smoothing) not only increases EFF but also minimises the differences between EFF determinations at different counting statistics. The parallelism between the curves of the individual patients persists

126

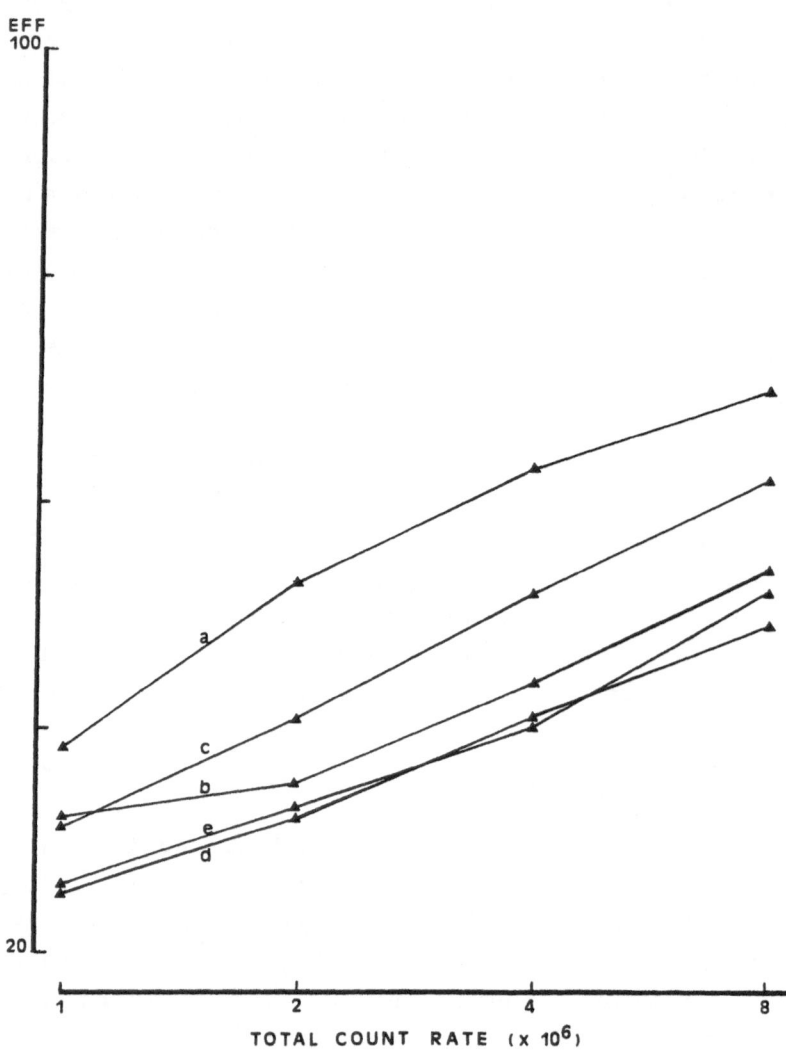

Fig. 50 . EFF determinations at different count rates. a,b,c,
d,e refer to 5 subjects with varying degree of RWMD.

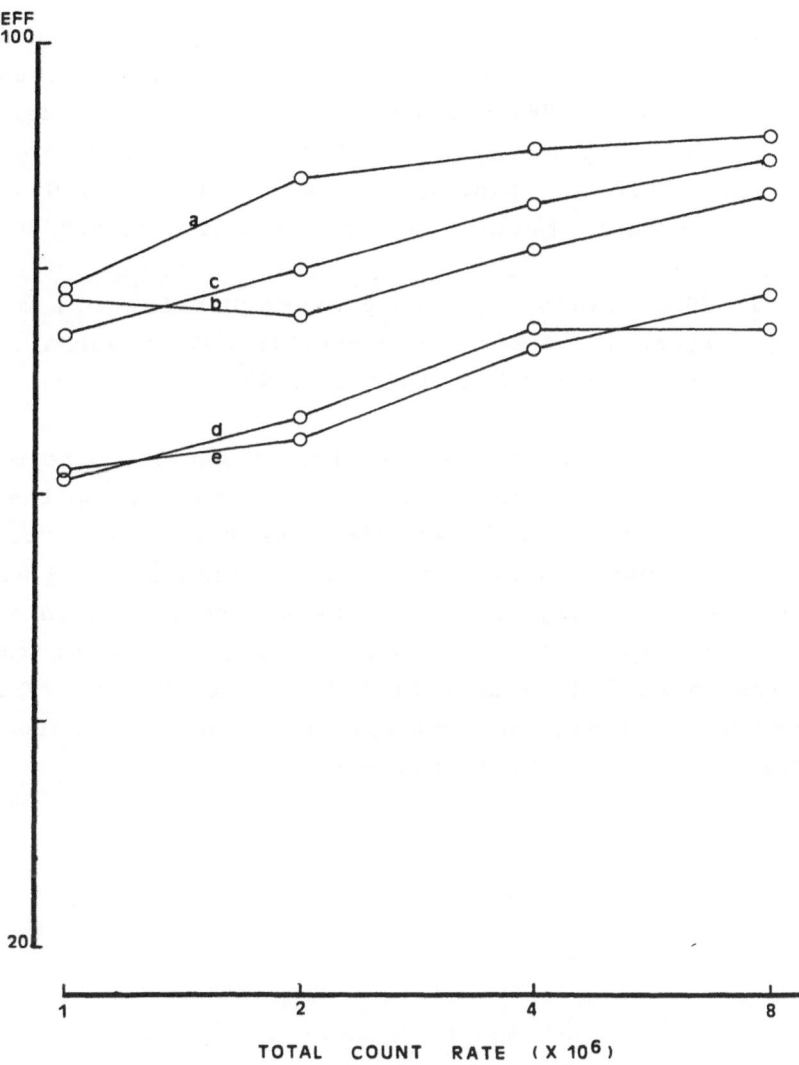

Fig. 51. EFF determinations after preprocessing of raw data.
a,b,c,d,e, refer to the same patients as in Fig. 2.

10.2.3.  <u>Normal values</u>,  <u>reproducibility</u>,  <u>effect of patient</u>
         <u>position</u>.

In a test group of 15 EGNA studies performed as
described in 4.2.in patients without heart disease we
determined LVCI, LVFI and LVEff within a manually delineated
left ventricular ROI. mean LVCI was 95.7 %, s.d. 1.39; mean
LVFI was 94.8 %,   s.d. 2.27;  mean LVEff was 91.5, s.d.
2.36. In the same group mean LVEF was 62.8 %, s.d. 8.6.

In 20 patients EGNA was performed twice in a modified
LAO position. The inter assay coefficient of variation was:
LVCI: 1.36%, LVFI: 1.62%, LVEff: 2.89%.

As in theory the effect of non tangential abnormalities
in contractility would be weakened as compared to the effect
of tangentially localised disturbances, we studied the
effect of position on the CI measurements in 15 patients
with a wide variety of RWMD. EGNA was performed in anterior
and in modified LAO position. The ROI was drawn manually
always to include both ventricles. Mean CI was 77.6 % for
anterior acquisitions and 75.6 % in LAO. The inter assay
variation coefficient became 4.1%.

10.3. CLINICAL STUDIES

10.3.1. Severity of RWMD

The relationship between the indices under resting conditions and the severity of RWMD was evaluated in a group of 97 patients with significant CAD on coronary arteriography. The patients were classified according to the findings on contrast ventriculography into 3 categories: absence of RWMD, presence of 1 or more localised hypo or akinetic segments, presence of 1 or more dyskinetic segments. The statistical significance between the values observed for the 3 groups was analysed using a Mann-Whitney U test.

All 3 indices decreased significantly (p<.0003) with increasing wall motion disturbances (fig.52). In the absence of RWMD, the values did not differ from those observed in normal individuals.

Figure 53 represents the relationship between the decrease in CI and FI resulting from RWMD. There exists only a poor correlation between both variables especially in the group of patients with hypokinesis where the decrease in FI is more severe than the decrease in CI.

130

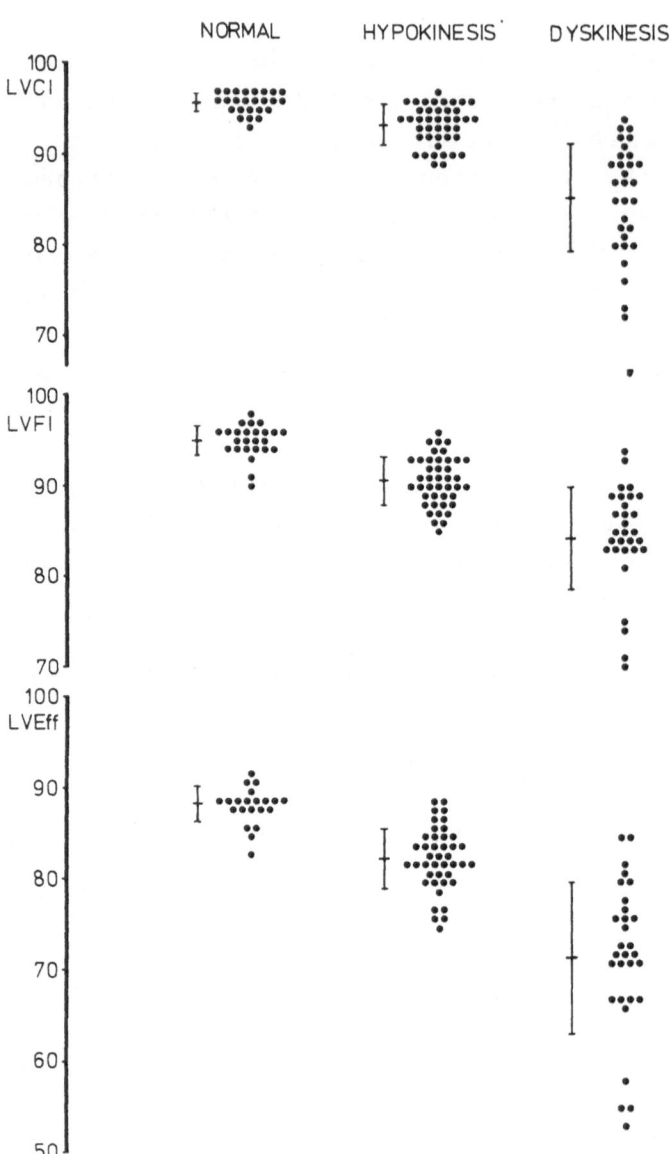

Fig.52. Relationship between the indices and the severity of RWMD

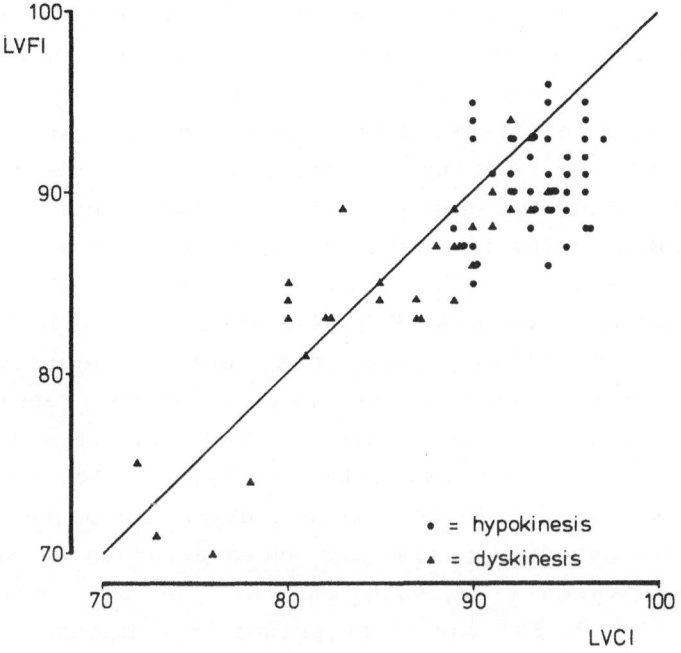

Fig. 53. Relationship between the decrease in CI and FI
resulting from RWMD.

## 10.3.2. Relationship between global and regional ventricular function during exercise testing

Submaximal exercise EGNA was performed in supine position as previously described (Chapter 6). The study group consisted of 3 normal individuals and 31 patients with proven CAD. The left ventricular response to exercise was analysed by means of the following parameters: relative variations in mBP, HR, EDV, SV and CI. The relative variations in EDV, SV as well as in LVEF were measured from nett LV time/activity curves calculated after correction of the original averaged cardiac cycle for unstructured background by uniform thresholding. Only rest/exercise data of comparable statistical noise were taken into account. mBP was calculated as 1/3 systolic BP + 2/3 diastolic BP.

No single relationship between the variations in CI and LVEF was evidenced during exercise. We therefore applied a principle component analysis (using the Fortran program package SIMCA 2T (8) to the whole data set. The structure of the data set was analysed by the use of 2 dimensional eigenvector projections (Fig.54). It can be seen that the data set is not homogeneous but that it consists of 2 separate clusters. One of them was exclusively composed of patients with triple vessel disease and anterior wall motion disturbances at exercise: patients 19, 14, 18, 20, 9, 17. The extreme patients in the other cluster had posterior wall motion disturbances, in some instances extended to the right ventricle: patients 23, 4, 6, 21. The 3 normal individuals were: 38, 40, 41. For the first principle component axis the variables which contributed most (with decreasing weight) were: EDV, CI and HR; CI and HR having a positive contribution in this direction, whereas EDV had a negative contribution. The most contributing variables in the second principle component axis axis were, with decreasing weight: SV (-), BP (+), HR (+) and CI (-).

133

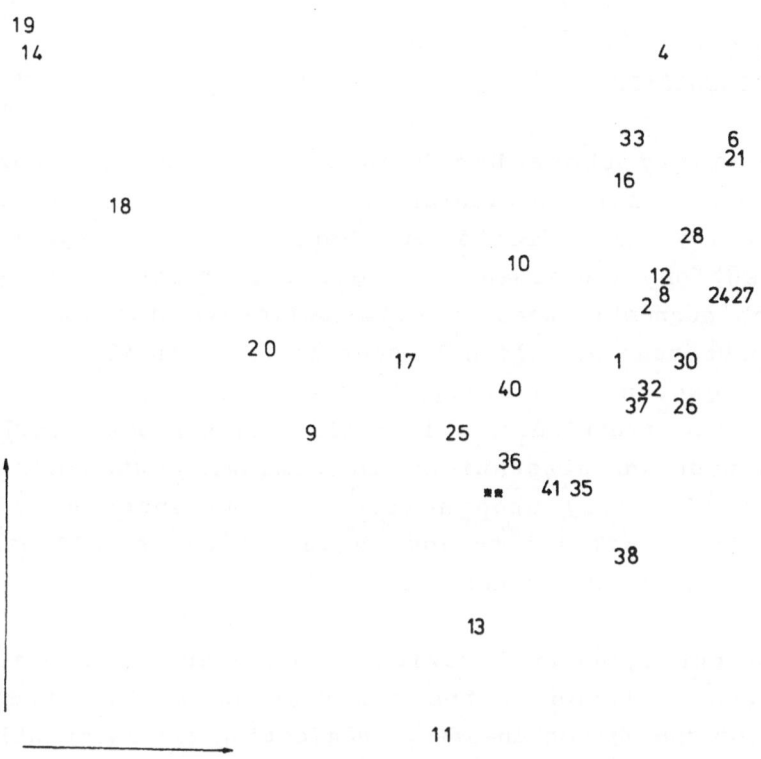

Fig. 54. Eigenvector projection of the autoscaled exercise
data set: first eigenvector (horizontal) versus
second eigenvector (vertical).

A tentative physiopathological interpretation of these data might be that the most affected patients in the first subgroup are characterised by an increase in EDV and a decrease in the synchronism of ventricular contraction in response to the increased demands on cardiac output. The most affected patients in the other subgroup cannot increase sufficiently their SV, whilst their mBP and HR increase and whilst the synchronism of ventricular contraction decreases.


10.4. DISCUSSION

Recently there has been an increasing effort to quantify regional ventricular dysfunction in order to assess objectively the effects of therapeutic or physiologic interventions and disease on ventricular performance. One approach currently used in radionuclide ventriculography is the measurement of regional ejection fraction (9, 10). While this procedure adequately documents alterations in the magnitude of ventricular wall motion, it neglects nearly all information on alterations in timing. Furthermore, EF measurements rely upon an accurate measurement of end diastolic volume and to some extent they are affected by preload and afterload conditions (11).

In our approach, regional ventricular function is described in terms of the combination of magnitude and timing of the volume changes, neglecting all information on absolute volume. In contrast to first harmonic amplitude/phase analysis, the indices described here overcome the problems of modelisation as the real count rate changes are used for calculation. The poor correlation between the decrease in CI and FI resulting from RWMD demonstrates that the accuracy of a temporal model limited to the first harmonic is a function of cardiac function itself.

The measurement of indices of ventricular function related to end diastolic volume requires that one accounts for activity generated by non ventricular structures, a problem which is not trivial (12). The calculation of minimum and maximum images offers a unique solution. In principle, the reproducibility of CI, FI and Eff measurements is only affected by the delineation of the left ventricle and by the projection used for the acquisition. Their usefulness is restricted, however, by the fact that they were experimentally found to be strongly dependent on counting statistics. This limits their clinical applicability to studies performed within relatively narrow limits of count rate.

Within the left ventricle, regional volume changes during the cardiac cycle result from electrical activation, myocardial contraction and passive movements and valve function. Disturbances in one of these factors will determine the ultimate value of CI, FI and Eff as they may induce asynchronisms in regional volume changes. Although hypokinetic wall motion disturbances that do not induce an asynchronism in the regional volume changes cannot be differentiated from normal wall motion by our approach, in clinical situations we found a close correlation between the severity of RWMD described roentgenologically and CI, FI and Eff. In the presence of localised hypokinetic segments, FI might be a more sensitive index than CI. This probably corresponds to other observations, that a decreased relaxation velocity is the most sensitive sign of CAD (13). Since CAD is a localised disorder with respect to the myocardial walls, a standardised quantification of the regional wall motion response to exercise is an essential requirement to determine cardiovascular function more exhaustively. In patients without heart disease, CI is not significantly affected by the complex interventions on preload and afterload that occur during hemodialysis (1).

Analysis of the heart as a pump has been clinically centered upon the Frank Starling relation between EDV of the ventricle and its stroke volume. In this context, evaluation of cardiac function by conventional indices such as LVEF, considers the ventricle as a black box with unknown internal structure but with given magnitudes of input and output. In contrast our description emphasises the anisotropic character of ventricular pump function. Eff is related to the efficiency of the heart defined as the ratio of the work performed by an "ideal" synchronous pump to the actual work performed by the asynchronous ventricle. CI and FI respectively describe decreases in pump efficiency due to asynchronisms in emptying and filling.

REFERENCES

1.  Bossuyt A., Deconinck F. 1981. Quantification of regional wall motion disturbances by means of radionuclide ventriculography. IEEE Computers in Cardiology 539.
2.  Bossuyt A. Deconinck F. 1982. Radionuclide indices of cardiac function related to structural ventricular disorders. In: Digital Imaging: Clinical Advances in Nuclear Medicine. Esser P. (Ed.) 207.
3.  Adam W.E., Bitter F. 1980. Advances in heart imaging. In: Medical Radionuclide Imaging II. IAEA-SM-247, 195.
4.  Bacharach S., Green M., Bonow R. et al. 1982. A method for Objective Evaluation of Functional Images. J. Nucl. Med. 23, 285.
5.  Byrom E., Pavel D., Meyer-Pavel C. 1981. Phase images of gated cardiac studies: A standard evaluation procedure. In: Functional Mapping of Organ Systems. Esser P.(Ed.) 129.
6.  Liehn J., Valeyre J., Collet E. et al. 1981. Etude de la cinetique ventriculaire regionale par representation dans le plan complexe. Proc. XXIIe Coll. de Med. Nucl. de Langue Franc. 55.
7.  Bacharach S., Green M. De Graaf C. et al. 1981. Fourier phase distribution maps in the left ventricle: toward an understanding of what they mean. In: Functional Mapping of Organ Systems. Esser P. (Ed.) 139.
8.  Albano C., Blomqvist G., Coomans D. et al. 1981. Pattern recognition by means of disjoint principle component models (SIMCA). Philosophy and Methods. Symposium i anvendt statistic. Denmarks Tekniske Hogskole 183.
9.  Maddox D.E., Holman B.L., Wyne J. et al. 1978. A noninvasive index of regional left ventricular wall motion. Am. J. Cardiol. 41, 1230.

10. Goris M.L., Briandet P.A., Huffer E. 1979. Automation and operator independent data processing of cardiac and pulmonary functions: role, methods and results. In: Information Processing in Medical Imaging. INSERM 88, 427.
11. Sonnenblick E.H., Strobeck J.E. 1977. Derived indexes of ventricular and myocardial function. New Eng. J.Med. 296, 978.
12. Goris M.L. 1979. Nontarget activities: can we correct for them? J. Nucl. Med. 20, 1312.
13. Bonow R.O., Bacharach S.L., Green M.F. 1981. Impaired ventricular diastolic filling in patients with coronary artery disease. Assessment with radionuclide ventriculography. Circulation. 64, 315.

CONCLUSIONS

A temporal Fourier transform (TFT) applied on a time series of scintigraphic images concentrates on the change in information contained in each picture element as a function of time. Basically it is a mathematical device that performs data extraction through data reduction of the activity/time relations present in the original data. An algorithm for the calculation on a pixel by pixel basis of the first harmonic amplitude and phase is easily implemented in a dedicated mini-computer for nuclear medicine. Both amplitude and phase are displayed as parametric functional images. In order to obtain a standard presentation of the results we developed a cyclic color scale, an essential requirement for the unequivocal display of the phase image. It then appears that, within the restrictions of the first harmonic as a temporal model for the process under study, a TFT allows a higher phase resolution than the actual sampling frequency of the original data.

The approximation of the impulse response by a sinusoidal function has no physiological counterpart when a TFT is applied to the study of transient phenomena such as superior vena caval imaging. Nevertheless as compared to conventional maximum and time of maximum images, the statistical value of the parametric images is improved. To study mediastinal flow obstruction induced by retrosternal goiters, superior cavography was performed with the neck in

extension and repeated with the neck in flexion.
Amplitude/phase images allowed to observe abnormal venous
flow patterns, changing with the neck position, and thus
suggesting the presence of mobile, non fixed and possibly
resectable lesions responsible for a superior vena cava
syndrome.

By means of dynamic lung transmission scintigraphy, the
periodic variations in density in the thorax during an
averaged respiratory cycle are recorded as digital
radiological images. The nowadays available detectors that
allow single photon counting yield only crude information
from the point of view of spatial resolution, but the
dynamic information in the data reflect the mechanical
effects of breathing. The application of the functional
imaging procedure to these data allowed to differentiate
normal from pathological states and to objectify the effect
of therapy in COPD patients.

The movement of the blood pool during an averaged
cardiac cycle observed in equilibrium gated nuclear
angiography (EGNA) is amenable to systematic analysis in
terms of amplitude and phase. The variations in blood volume
(space, time) are detected and recorded as 2 dimensional
projections of variations in count rate (image, time). The
original data are characterised by a high level of
structured background, stationary in time. The compression
of the relevant information on the temporal variations in
count rate into 2 parametric images overcomes some of the
limitations of the visual inspection of the EGNA studies due
to image contrast, photon noise and limited sampling
frequency. With respect to this, amplitude and phase images
compare favorably with other count rate derived functional
images. The accuracy of the model for the temporal behaviour
of the ventricular volume changes will depend on the
contribution of the first harmonic to the information

content of the whole Fourier spectrum. This holds also true for more sophisticated displays of the phase information.

Disturbances in regional myocardial contraction result in decreased and delayed blood volume movements. As such, the evaluation of regional wall motion disturbances in terms of magnitude and timing of the temporal variations in count rate relies upon a more fundamental aspect of the tracer technique rather than upon a pure morphological interpretation. This approach is conceptually different from the evaluation of RWMD by contrast ventriculography or by earlier scintigraphic techniques, which concentrate on the extension of the ventricular borders during systole. For a qualitative evaluation, the restriction to the first harmonic component of the activity changes allows a clinically adequate detection and localisation of RWMD, including those of the right ventricle.

The possibility of assessing RWMD non invasively allows a more extensive evaluation of regional myocardial contraction during intervention studies and in critically ill patients. The objectivation of RWMD during exercise radionuclide ventriculography proved to be more sensitive and more specific than ECG anomalies or Tl myocardial perfusion defects for the diagnosis of LAD or CX stenoses. The appearance of RWMD was not sensitive for the detection of RCA stenoses, although the observation of RWMD was very specific for the latter condition. During acute myocardial infarction we observed more severe alterations in the sequence of ventricular wall motion (as determined by the phase image) in patients with anterior than in patients with posterior myocardial infarction. In the early evolution of the infarction, the synchronism of the regional ventricular blood volume changes improved most in patients with posterior myocardial infarction. This improvement correlated with an improvement in global ventricular function as

determined by left ventricular ejection fraction. These
observations, suggesting functional dissimilarity of the
anterior and posterior walls, emphasize the necessity to
quantify the synchronism in regional ventricular blood
changes and to correlate regional ventricular motion to
global ventricular function in a standardised manner.

In patients with disturbances in electrical activation
of the ventricles, the phase image demonstrated marked
differences in both localisation and timing of the blood
pool movements. The characterisation of distinct phase
patterns for various types of intraventricular conduction
disturbances contributed largely to the interest raised by
phase analysis in the U.S.. Although the first harmonic
model does not allow to differentiate between timing
differences occuring during ventricular emptying or filling
periods, amplitude/phase analysis optimises the perception
of magnitude and timing of count rate changes to an extent
that cannot be observed by more conventional data processing
procedures.

Mathematically it can be demonstrated that as long as
amplitude/phase analysis is restricted to a first harmonic
model, the subdivision of the cardiac cycle in only 4 images
is sufficient for the calculation of the parametric images
by a temporal Hadamard transform. In selected clinical
situations, such as in patients with valvular disorders, the
inability to differentiate between alterations in emptying
or filling may introduce a lack of specificity of the
amplitude/phase patterns. As an alternative procedure, we
therefore developed a method of temporal contrast
enhancement, which in terms of Fourier analysis, conserves
all the Fourier frequencies of an averaged cardiac cycle
except the zero frequency component. Both the clinical
applicability of the temporal Hadamard transform and the
improved perception of timing differences by temporal

contrast enhancement relate the choice of pattern recognition procedures in clinical practice to psychophysical characteristics of human vision.

Within a first harmonic model, the effect of regional asynchronism on global ventricular performance can be evaluated as the amplitude of the regional variations in blood volume modulated by their phase. Extended to the whole frequency spectrum, we have defined 3 parameters which quantify ventricular pump function as the ratio of the efficient blood volume changes (stroke volume) to the actual blood volume changes occuring throughout the cardiac cycle as a result of asynchronisms in ventricular emptying or filling or both. By comparing the individual pumping contributions located at each pixel with the net result for the global pumping behaviour, these indices give an idea of the efficiency with which all parts of the ventricle cooperate in order to generate the desired pumping action. The practical usefulness of the indices, however, is restricted by the fact that they were found to be strongly dependent on counting statistics. Preliminary clinical investigations have shown the indices to be quite promising for assessing structural disturbances in ventricular function, with emphasis on the anisotropic character of the ventricular pump.

The investigation of amplitude/phase patterns in cardiac blood pool studies may be justified by the physical properties of the original data as determined by the acquisition procedure, the pathophysiological model of the process under study and the psychophysical characteristics of our perception. While the functional imaging procedure originally aimed at the conversion of the original data to images better suited for visual inspection, the interpretation of blood volume changes in terms of amplitude and phase resulted in the extraction of quantitative information on ventricular pump efficiency. In this context optimal function can be compromised by two types of local factors: the first is the presence of ventricular wall segments that do not contribute enough to the pumping action i.e. an amplitude defect. The second is a lack of synchronicity between various segments of the ventricular wall, i.e. timing defects. A description of the intraventricular blood pool movements in this way contrasts with conventional indices of cardiac status which generally define ventricular function in terms of magnitude of input and output. It is expected that, in the light of the complex cardiac morphology, the determination of asynergy indices will provide a clinical tool for further investigations into the relationships between structure and function.

# COLOR PLATES

COLOR PLATES

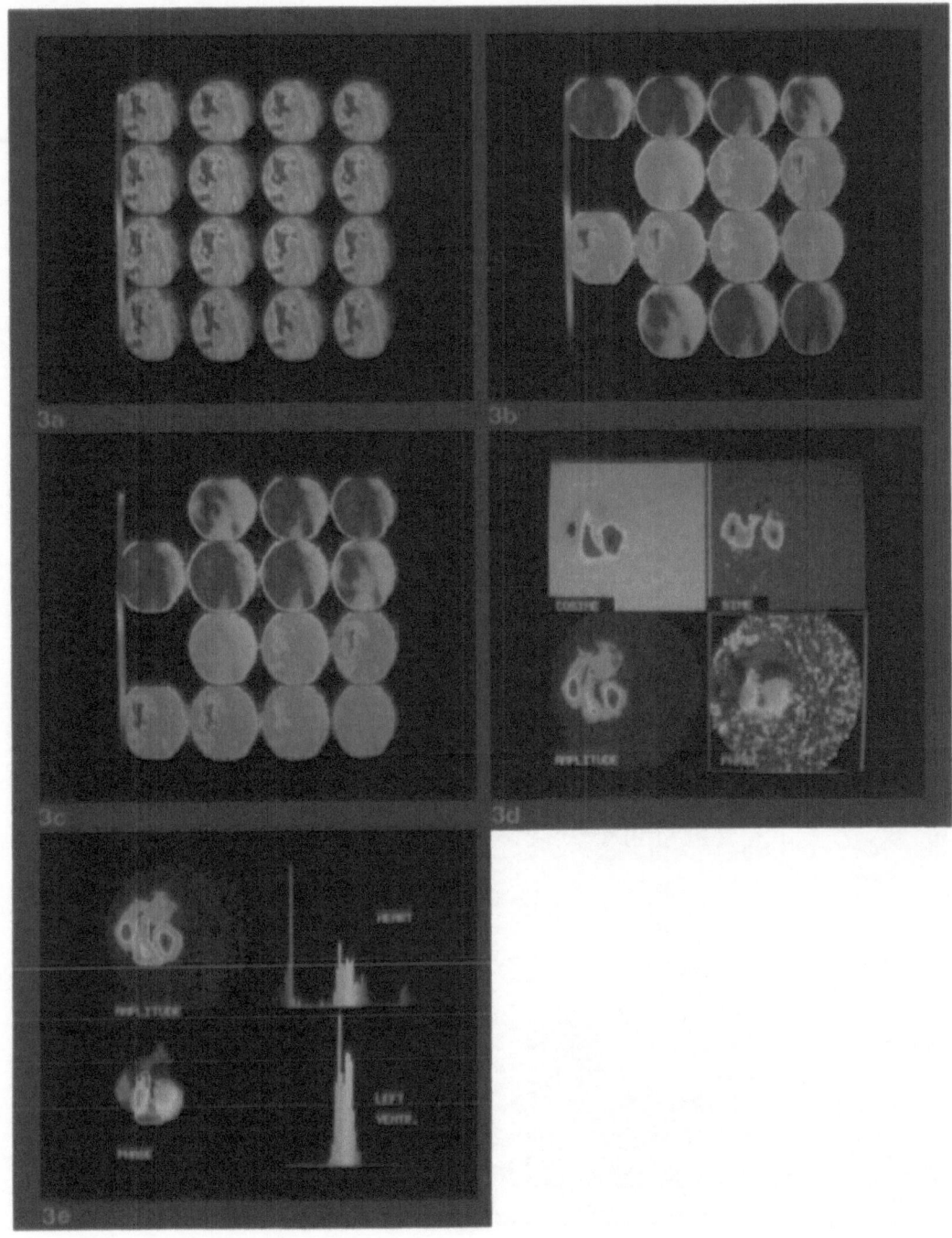

Fig. 3. Generation of amplitude and phase images of an equilibrium gated cardiac blood pool study

3.a. original data/3.b. cosine series/3.c. sine series/3.d. functional images/3.e. amplitude/phase images

148

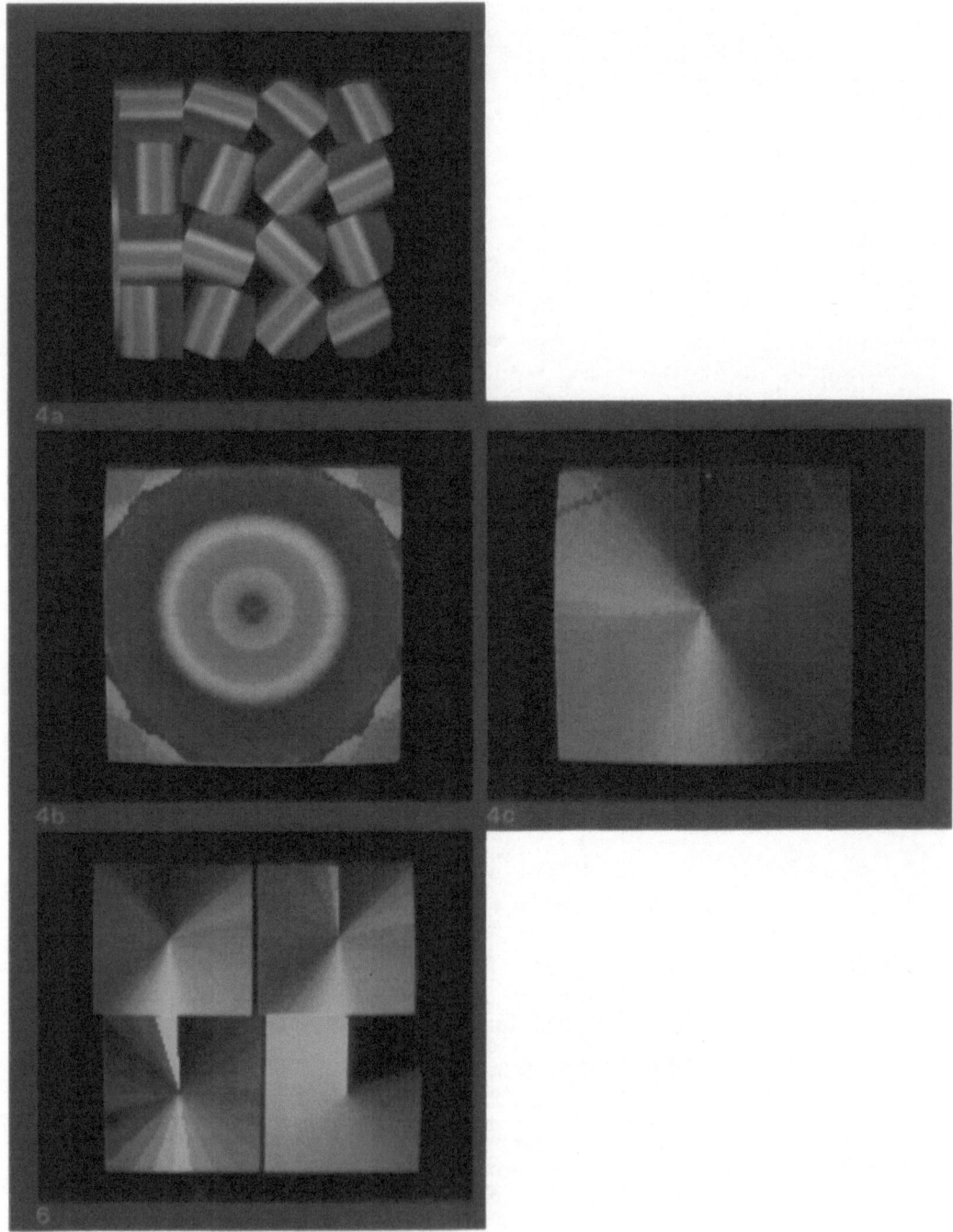

Fig. 4. Simulation study of a periodic phenomenon
    4.a. original data/4.b. linearly increasing amplitude/4.c. phase image in cyclic color code

Fig. 6. Representation of the phase image of Fig. 4.c. in different conventional color codes and in the cyclic color code

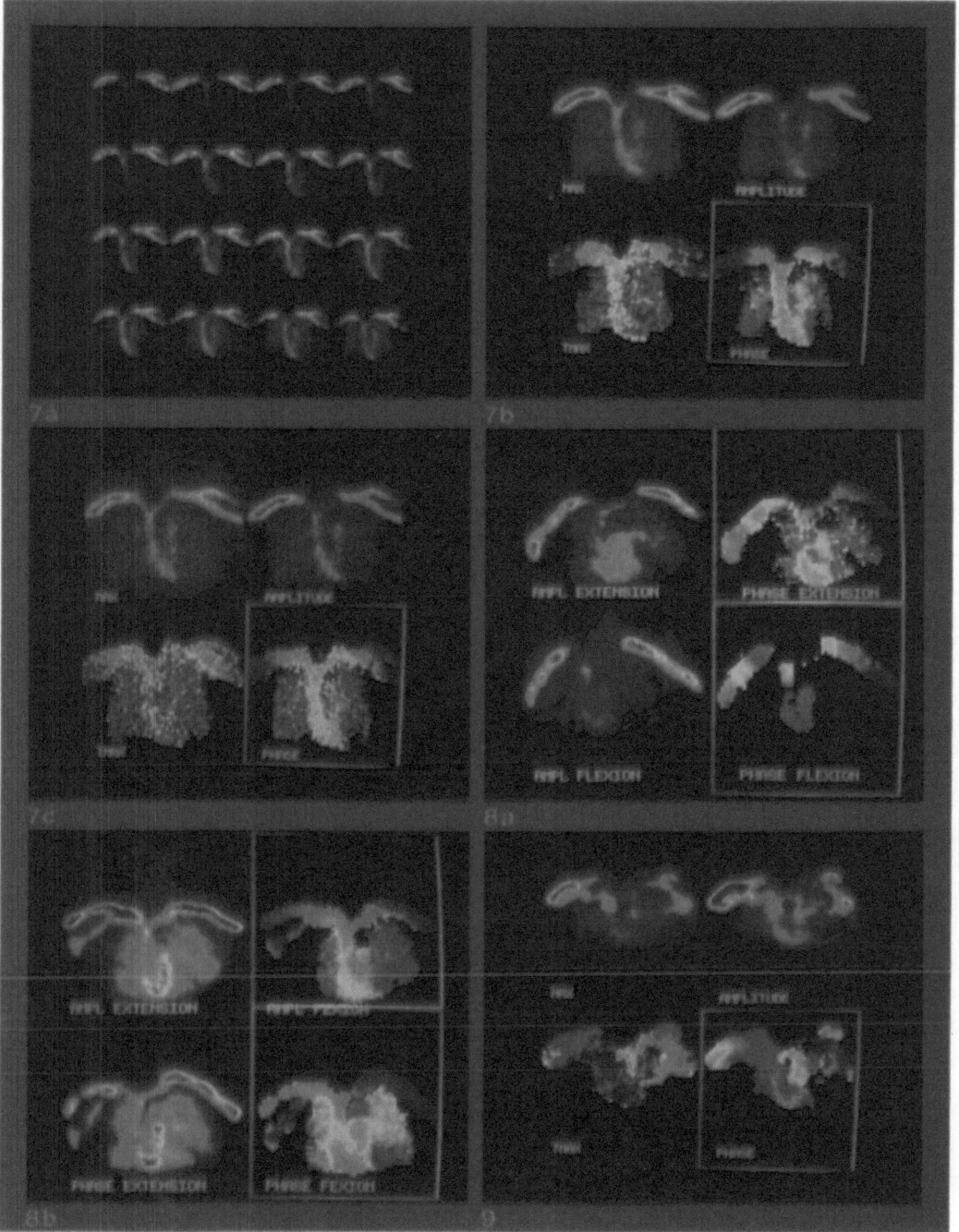

Fig. 7. Radionuclide superior cavography in a normal control subject
    7.a. preprocessed image series of tracer transit through mediastinum/7.b. functional images/7.c. functional images without preprocessing

Fig. 8. Fixed SVC syndrome in patient 1
    8.a. before thyroidectomy/8.b. one month after thyroidectomy

Fig. 9. Visualisation of collateral circulation on the functional images in patient 2

150

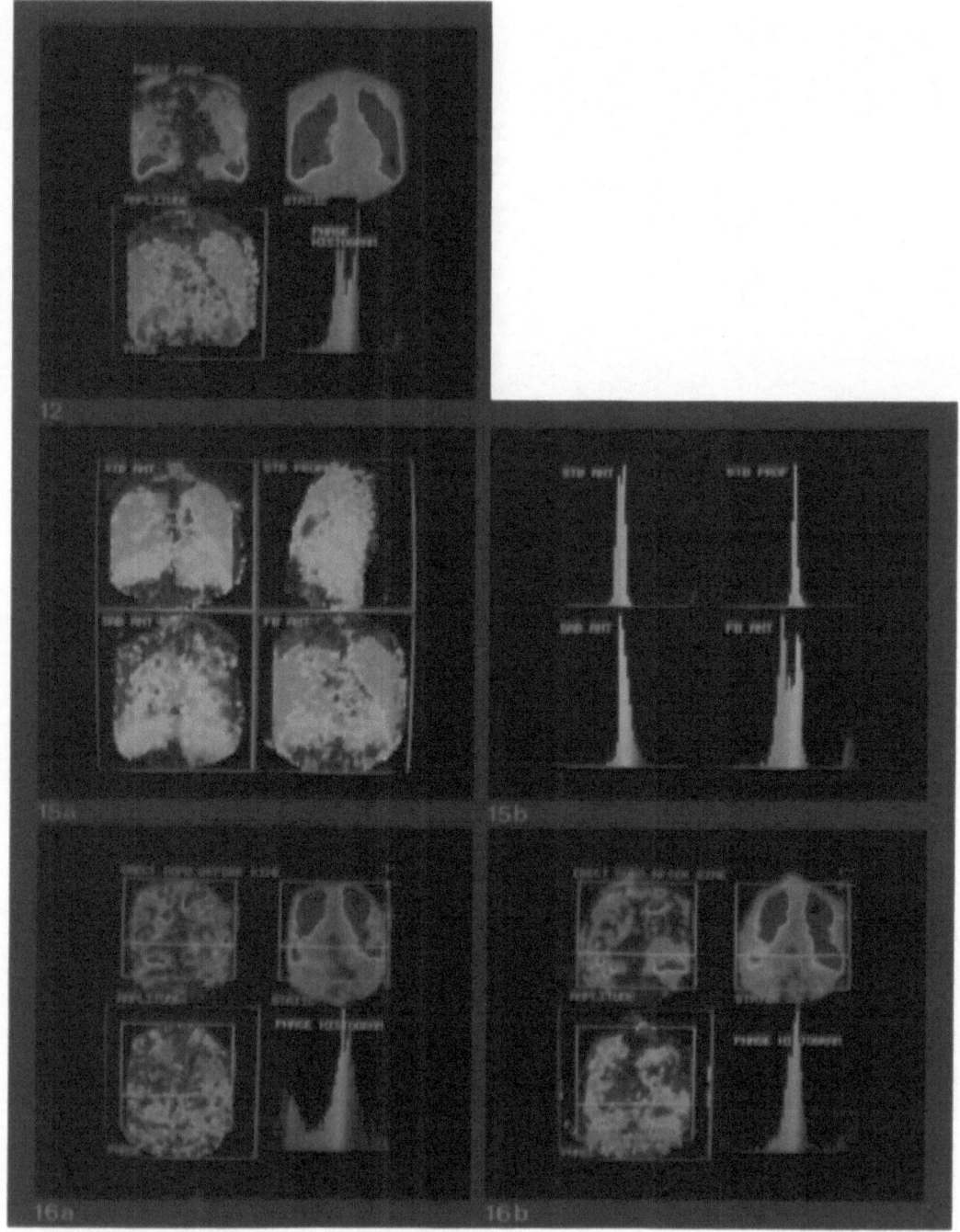

Fig. 12. Processed data series obtained during erect FB

Fig. 15. Phase images and amplitude/phase histograms with different breathing manoeuvres
  15.a. phase images/15.b. amplitude/phase histograms

Fig. 16. Transmission study in COPD patients
  16.a. before AAB retraining/16.b. after AAB retraining

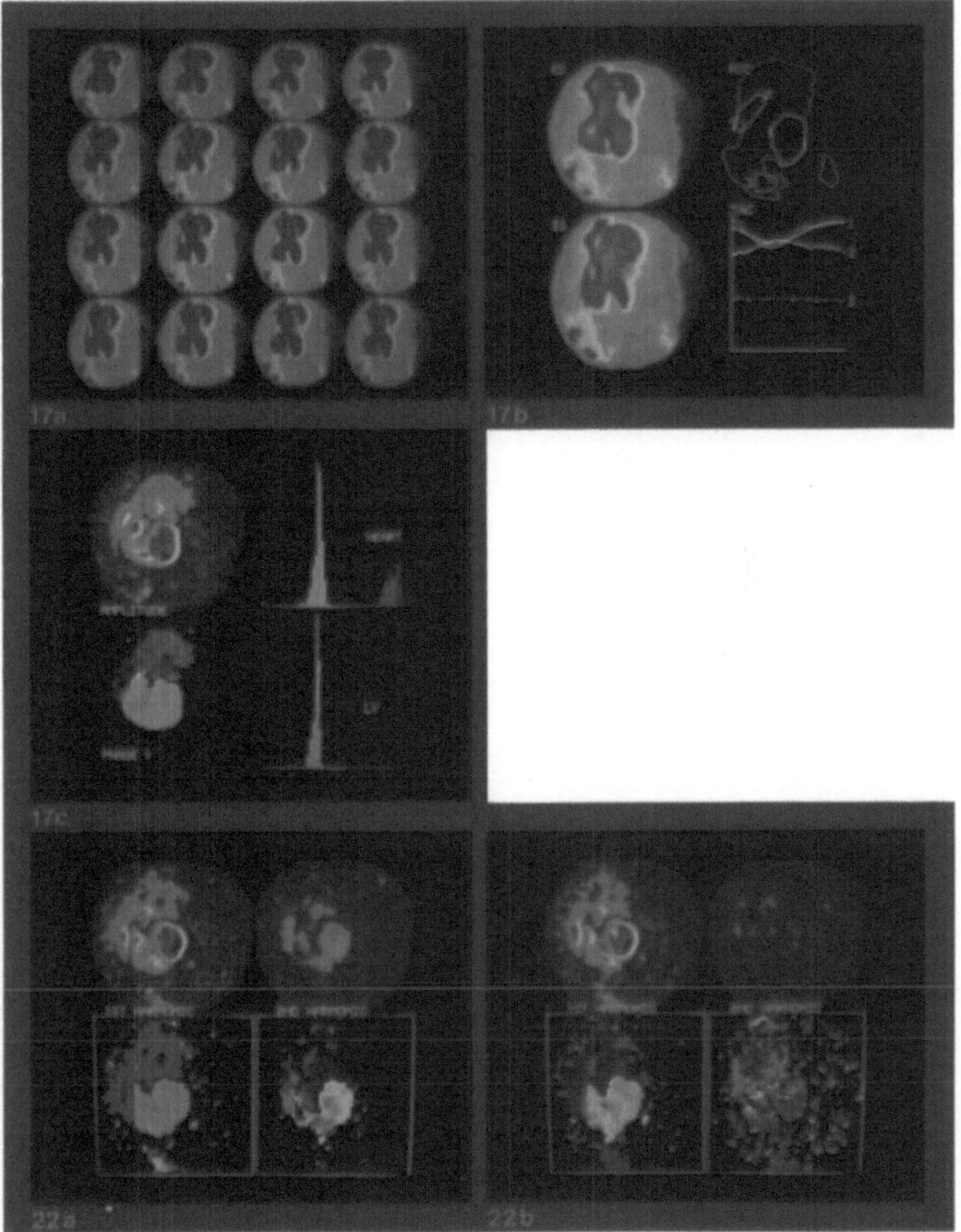

Fig. 17. EGNA study in a normal control person

    17.a. original (preprocessed) data series/17.b. ul : end diastolic frame; 11 : end systolic frame; ur : ROI over LV, RV, liver; lr : TAC + fitted sine functions/17.c. ul : amplitude image; 11 : phase image; ur : amplitude/phase distribution in global image; lr : amplitude/phase distribution in LV

Fig. 22. Effect of cycle length on 1st and 2nd harmonic amplitude and phase images in a patient with a long diastasis period. 2nd Harmonic amplitude is scaled to maximum of 1st harmonic amplitude

    22.a. basic frequency = heart frequency / 22 b diastasis period discarded.

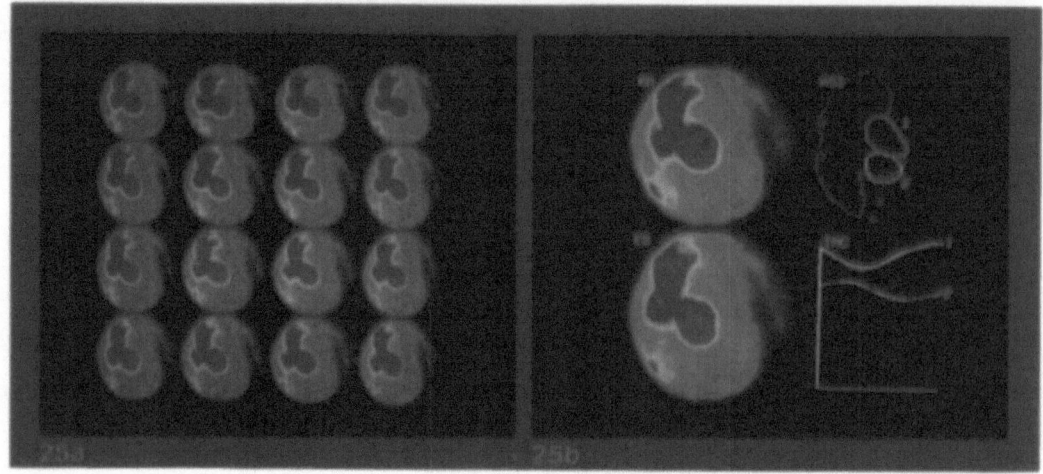

Fig. 25. EGNA study in a patient with an antero-apical aneurysm
    25.a. original(preprocessed) data series/25.b. ul : end diastolic frame; 11: end
systolic frame; ur : ROI 1 and ROI 2; lr : TAC + fitted sine functions

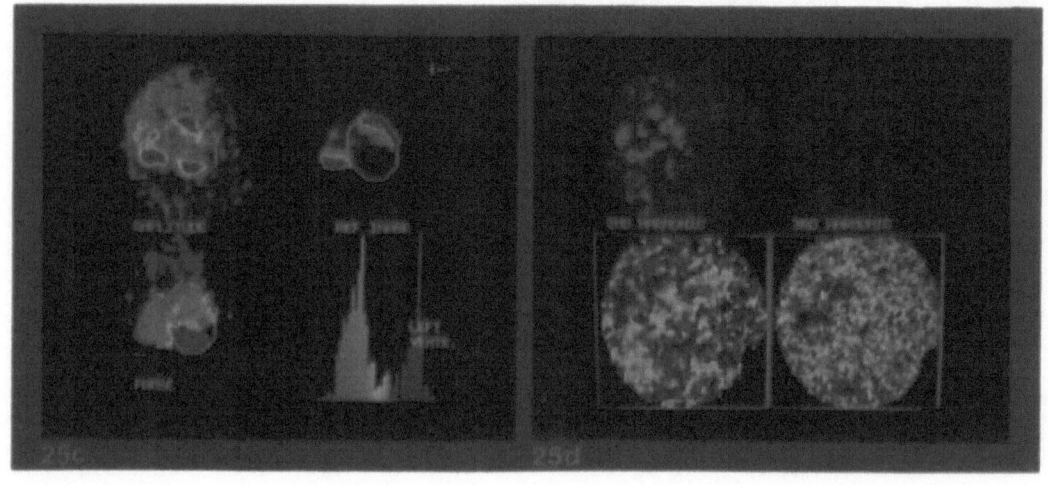

25.c. ul : amplitude image; 11 : phase image; ur : REF image; lr : LV amplitude/phase distribution/
25.d. higher harmonic images

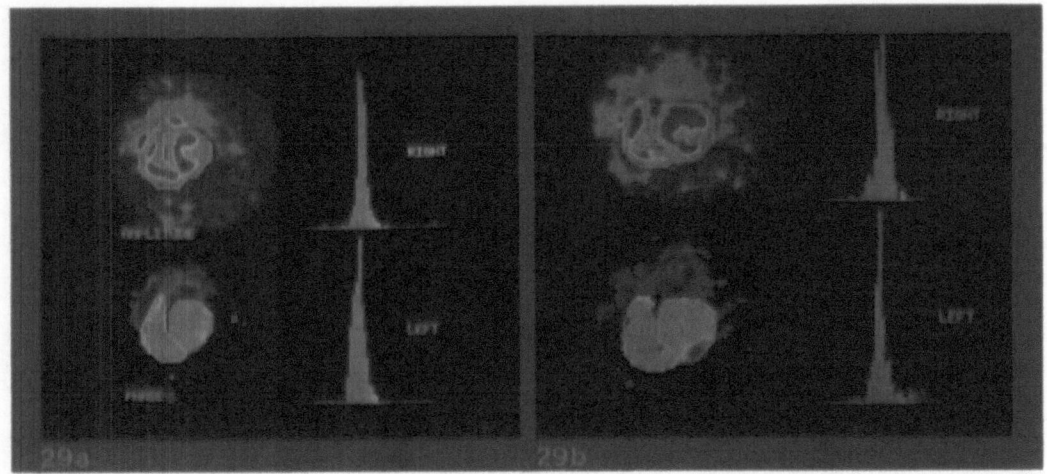

Fig. 29. Examples of RWMD with increasing severity and different localisations
29.a. posterolateral hypokinesis/29.b. posterobasal dyskinesis

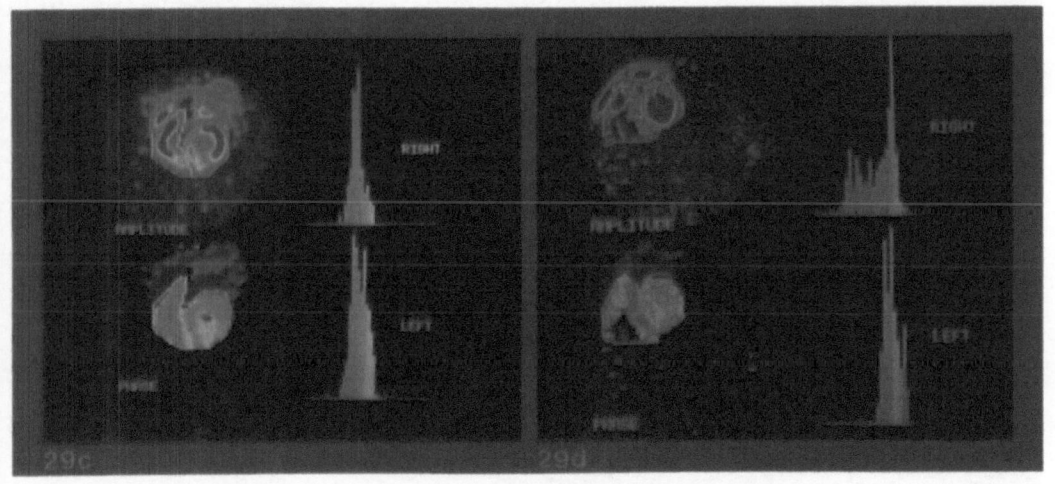

29.c. anterior dyskinesis/29.d. right ventricular dyskinesis

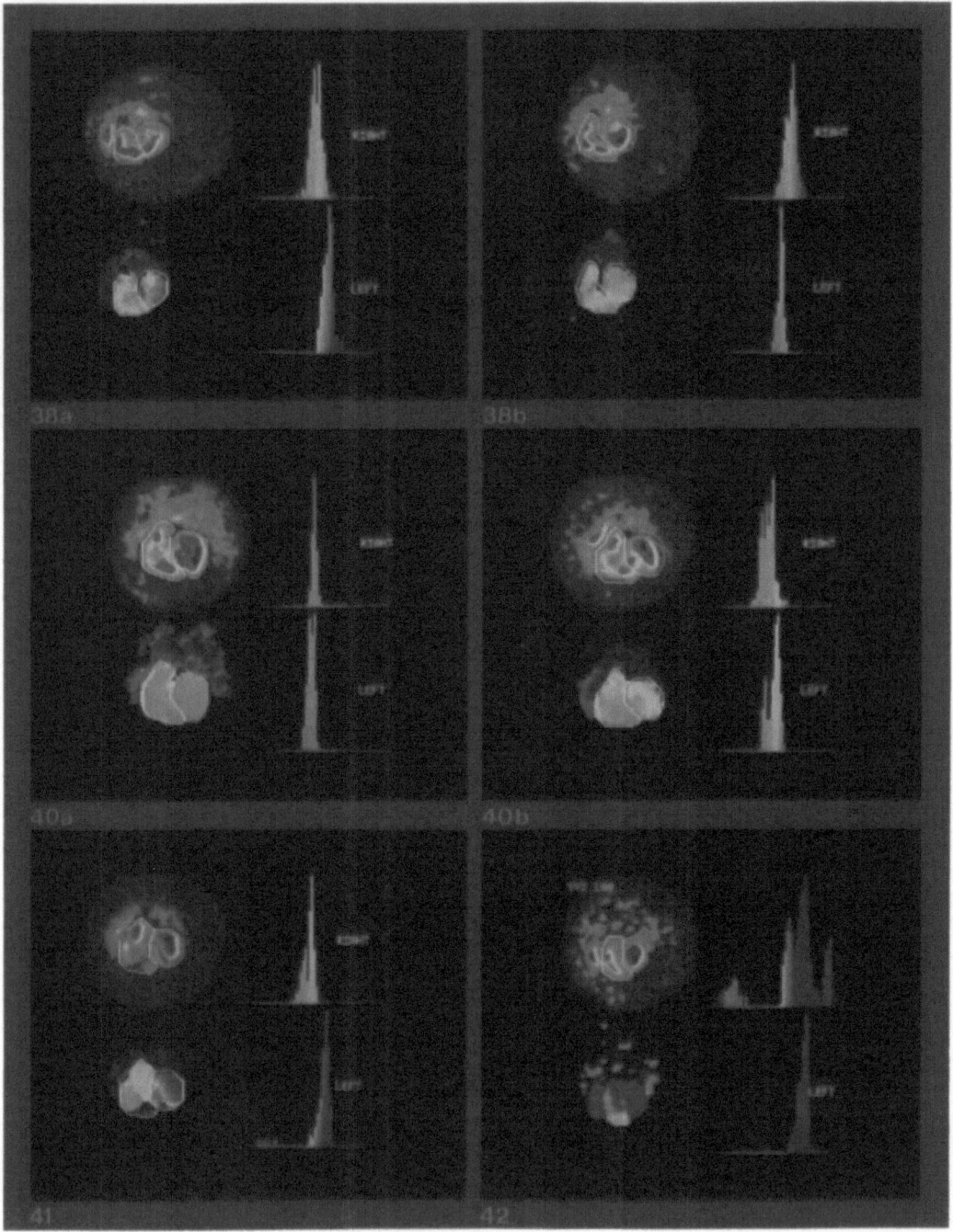

Fig. 38. Typical amplitude/phase distribution
   38.a. in LBBB/38.b. in RBBB

Fig. 40. Effect of pace maker stimulation
   40.a. normal sinus rhythm/40.b. RV pace maker stimulation 70/min.

Fig. 41. Effect of ventricular pacing at high frequencies

Fig. 42. Effect of retrograde atrial activiation

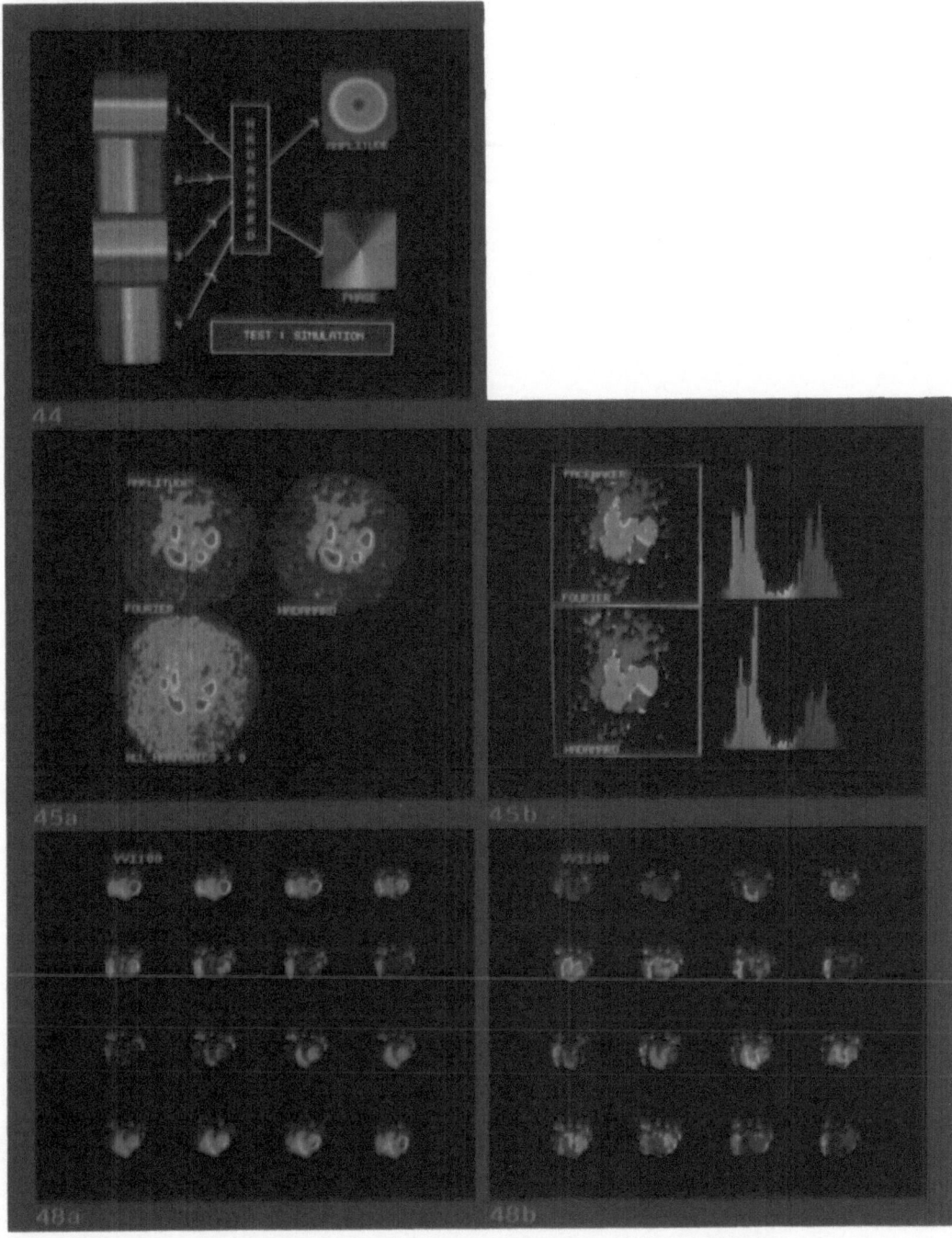

Fig. 44 Application of Hadamard transform to simulation study of periodic phenomenon

Fig. 45. Comparison of Fourier and Hadamard transform in EGNA study of a patient with RV pace maker stimulation at 120/min.

45.a. amplitude information/45.b. phase information

Fig. 48. Temporal contrast enhancement and fractional variation image series of EGNA study in a patient with retrograde atrial activation during VVI pacing

48.a. temporal contrast enhancement/48.b. fractional variation image series

# INDEX OF SUBJECTS

Acute myocardial infarction: 86-99, 103
Aortic stenosis: 115
Augmented abdominal breathing: 37-41
Bolus progression images: 27
Breathing patterns: 33-41
Bundle branch blocks: 101-108
CAD identification: 70-85
Conduction disturbances: 101-108
Contrast ventriculography: 62, 129
COPD: 37-41
Cyclic color scale: 16, 18, 46
Effect of noice: 44-53, 125-127
EGNA (principle): 43-45
Exercise testing: 70-83, 132
Factor analysis: 4
First harmonic model: 12, 49, 53, 108, 112, 118
First pass studies: 15, 20-27
Fourier analysis (principle): 5, 9-19, 113
Fractional variation imaging: 116
Frank Starling mechanism: 98, 136
Gating artefacts: 51
Hadamard transform: 110-114, 117
Higher harmonics: 13, 49-54, 59, 119, 123
Isotopic cavography: 20
Left ventricular ejection fraction: 88-99
Lung transmission scintigraphy: 29-41
Mitral valve prosthesis: 115
Onset of mechanical systole: 107
Pace maker stimulation: 104-108
Periodic phenomena, simulation: 11, 14
Phase distribution function: 18, 121

Phase distribution histogram: 18, 36-39, 58, 101
Preprocessing: 2, 22, 32, 45, 51-52, 127
Principle component analysis: 4, 132
Regional stroke volume: 49
Regional ejection fraction: 49
Response function: 4, 5,20 27, 138
Retrograde ventriculo atrial conduction:106
Right ventricle dysfunction: 61, 78, 93
Rose's formalism: 118
RWMD:
    in AMI: 92-99
    interpretation:56-68
    localisation: 59, 63-68, 74, 102
    quantification: 121, 129-131
Stress ECG: 72,75
Superior vena cava syndrome: 21-28
Synergy indices: 122-136
Temporal contrast enhancement: 115-119
Tl myocardial scintigraphy: 73, 75